T0192707

Hematopathology and Coagulation

Hematopathology and Coagulation

Self-Assessment and Board Review

Amer Wahed, M.D.
Associate Professor, Department of Pathology
University of Texas Health Science Center, Houston, TX, USA

Jesse Manuel Jaso, M.D.
Assistant Professor, Department of Pathology
University of Texas Southwestern Medical Center, Dallas, TX, USA

Ashok Tholpady, M.D.
Assistant Professor, Department of Pathology and Laboratory Medicine
University of Texas MD Anderson Cancer Center, Houston, TX, USA

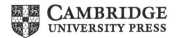
CAMBRIDGE
UNIVERSITY PRESS

CAMBRIDGE
UNIVERSITY PRESS

University Printing House, Cambridge CB2 8BS, United Kingdom

One Liberty Plaza, 20th Floor, New York, NY 10006, USA

477 Williamstown Road, Port Melbourne, VIC 3207, Australia

314-321, 3rd Floor, Plot 3, Splendor Forum, Jasola District Centre, New Delhi - 110025, India

79 Anson Road, #06-04/06, Singapore 079906

Cambridge University Press is part of the University of Cambridge.

It furthers the University's mission by disseminating knowledge in the pursuit of
education, learning and research at the highest international levels of excellence.

www.cambridge.org
Information on this title: www.cambridge.org/9781316505601
DOI: 10.1017/9781316527429

First published 2017

A catalogue record for this publication is available from the British Library

Library of Congress Cataloging in Publication data
Names: Wahed, Amer, author. | Jaso, Jesse Manuel, author. | Tholpady, Ashok, author.
Title: Hematopathology and coagulation: self-assessment and board review /
Amer Wahed, Jesse Manuel Jaso, Ashok Tholpady.
Description: Cambridge; New York, NY: Cambridge University Press, 2017. |
Includes bibliographical references and index.
Identifiers: LCCN 2017007132 | ISBN 9781316505601 (paperback)
Subjects: | MESH: Hematologic Diseases – pathology | Hematology – methods | Examination Questions
Classification: LCC RB145 | NLM WH 18.2 | DDC 616.1/50076–dc23
LC record available at https://lccn.loc.gov/2017007132

ISBN 978-1-316-50560-1 Paperback

....

Contents

Preface

This book is designed as a self-assessment tool for individuals preparing for US and UK boards in clinical pathology and hematopathology.

Each chapter contains a mixture of common tested topics as well as more challenging ones. We recommend that readers who already have a reasonable grasp of the hematopathology topics use this book as a self-assessment tool. The book is conveniently divided into different chapters with answers and discussions at the end of each chapter.

We hope that candidates who are preparing for exams will find this a useful resource.

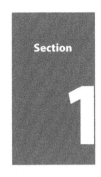

Non-Neoplastic Hematology

RBC Disorders

Hematopoiesis: Questions 1–14

1. The following are features of normal erythropoiesis except:
   A. Immature erythropoietic cells tend to form clusters which surround macrophages
   B. Proerythroblasts are large cells with deep blue cytoplasm with large nuclei and nucleoli
   C. Erythropoiesis occurs predominantly in the paratrabecular areas
   D. Reticulocytes typically have a three-day life span, of which two days are spent in the bone marrow

2. Which of the following is an effective marker for erythroid precursors?
   A. CD34
   B. CD71
   C. CD41
   D. CD61

3. Which of the following step is the rate-limiting step for heme biosynthesis?
   A. Formation of δ aminolevulinic acid from glycine and succinyl CoA
   B. Formation of prophobilinogen from δ aminolevulinic acid
   C. Formation of heme from protoporphyrin IX
   D. None of the above

4. Regarding granulopoiesis, which is true:
   A. Secondary granules are seen only at the band and mature granulocyte stage
   B. Blasts, promyelocytes and myelocytes all have nucleoli
   C. Granulopoiesis in a normal marrow is seen adjacent to bone
   D. Metamyelocytes are capable of cell division

5. Regarding erythropoiesis, which is true:
   A. All normoblasts have nucleoli
   B. The basophilic normoblast is the largest cell
   C. Erythropoiesis occurs in islands close to the bony trabecula
   D. The normal sequence of maturation is proerythroblast to basophilic normoblast to polychromatic normoblast to orthochromatic normoblast to reticulocyte to a mature red cell

6. Regarding megakaryopoiesis and megakaryocytes, which is true:
   A. Normal development of megakaryocytes is regulated by multiple cytokines and one principal one is thrombopoietin
   B. Clustering of megakaryocytes is a normal phenomenon
   C. Megakaryocytes mature through endomitosis where cell division with nuclear division occurs
   D. Megakaryocytes may cause destruction of hematopoietic cells by emperipolesis

7. Which of the following cell is derived from a hematopoietic stem cell?
   A. Osteoblasts
   B. Osteocytes
   C. Chondrocytes
   D. Osteoclasts

8. Features characteristic of erythroid precursors include all of the following except:
   A. In a normal marrow they are found as distinctive islands
   B. They adhere tightly to one another
   C. Cytoplasm is deep blue in the erythroblasts
   D. Shrinkage artifact of cytoplasm is seen in plastic-embedded sections

9. Regarding granulopoiesis:
   A. Both myelocytes and metamyelocytes are capable of cell division
   B. By light microscopy, promyelocytes of the three granulocytic lineages can easily be distinguished
   C. Myeloblasts are typically found in the paratrabecular areas and close to arterioles
   D. Indented myeloid cells are known as bands

10. Regarding megakaryopoiesis, which is true:
    A. Megakaryocytes are normally found close to bony trabeculae
    B. Normal megakaryocytes engulf and destroy hematopoietic cells
    C. Megakaryocytes undergo endomitosis (aka endoreduplication)
    D. Normal megakaryocyte nuclei have multiple distinct lobes

11. Which agents are responsible for the stimulation of eosinophils?
    A. IL-3
    B. IL-5
    C. GM-CSF
    D. All of the above

12. Secondary granules of neutrophils:
    A. Contain lactoferrin
    B. Are also known as azurophilic granules
    C. Contain peroxidase
    D. Are found in immature granulocytic cells

13. All of the following regarding erythropoiesis are true except:
    A. The life span of a mature erythrocyte is about four months
    B. On average each erythroblast forms eight reticulocytes
    C. In acute anemia, when accelerated erythropoiesis occurs, the red cells that are released into the circulation are normocytic and all bear the i antigen
    D. The mean time from the proerythroblast stage to reticulocyte is approximately five days

14. Regarding megakaryopoiesis and megakaryocytes:
    A. Megakaryocytes are approximately 10% of hematopoietic cells in a normal bone marrow
    B. Each megakaryocyte gives rise to 1,000–3,000 platelets
    C. Mature megakaryocytes contain 2N–128 N of DNA
    D. Mature megakaryocytes have little basophilic cytoplasm

CBC, Peripheral Smear and Bone Marrow Examination: Questions 15–40

15. When compared to normal adult CBC values, normal values for neonates and children differ considerably with the exception of:
    A. RBC count
    B. WBC count
    C. Platelet count
    D. Hemoglobin level

16. The following are true for hemoglobin measurement by automated analyzers:
    A. The red cells are required to be lysed
    B. The spectrophotometric method is typically used
    C. Absorbance of light at 540 nm is measured
    D. All of the above

17. Which of the following is a true statement?
    A. In oxyhemoglobin, iron is in the ferrous state
    B. In methemoglobin, iron is in the ferrous state
    C. In both oxyhemoglobin and methemoglobin, iron is in the ferrous state
    D. None of the above

18. Causes of falsely elevated hemoglobin levels by the spectrophotometric method include all of the following except:
    A. Leukocytosis
    B. Paraproteinemia
    C. Hyperlipidemia
    D. Thrombocytosis

19. Which of the following equations is correct to calculate MCH values?
    A. MCH= Hb/Hct
    B. MCH=Hb/RBC count
    C. MCH=Hb/MCV
    D. None of the above

20. One indication for warming the blood and repeating the CBC test is elevated:
    A. Hemoglobin
    B. Hct
    C. MCH
    D. MCHC

21. When the uncorrected WBC count is higher than the corrected WBC count, the most likely cause is:
    A. Presence of nucleated RBCs
    B. Presence of large platelets
    C. High lymphocyte count
    D. Presence of paraproteinemia

22. Causes of false low platelet count (pseudothrombocytopenia) include all of the following except:
    A. EDTA-induced platelet clumps
    B. EDTA-induced platelet satellitism
    C. Fragmented red cells
    D. Traumatic venepuncture

23. When a peripheral smear slide appears blue to the naked eye, a likely possibility is:
    A. Underlying chronic myeloproliferative disorder
    B. Underlying acute leukemia
    C. Underlying hemolytic anemia
    D. Underlying monoclonal gammopathy

24. A bone marrow exam reveals increased promyelocytes with paucity of more mature cells. Differential diagnosis includes:
    A. Acute promyelocytic leukemia
    B. Kostmann's syndrome
    C. Sepsis in a patient with agranulocytosis
    D. All of the above

25. The following are established causes of bone marrow granulomas:
    A. Hodgkin lymphoma
    B. Metastatic disease
    C. Histoplasmosis
    D. All of the above

26. Macrophages with "wrinkled tissue paper" appearance of the cytoplasm may be seen in all of the following conditions except:
    A. Gaucher's disease
    B. Niemann-Pick disease

C. Chronic myelogenous leukemia
    D. Sickle cell disease

27. Characteristic features of sea blue histicoytes that may be seen in bone marrow include:
    A. Yellow-brown macrophages with Giemsa stain
    B. Blue-green appearance with H&E stain
    C. They are macrophages containing ceroid
    D. They are PAS negative

28. Causes of a dry tap when performing a bone marrow aspiration may be expected in:
    A. Iron deficiency anemia
    B. Refractory anemia with ringed sideroblasts
    C. Hairy cell leukemia
    D. Hereditary spherocytosis

29. Regarding lymphoid infiltrates in the bone marrow:
    A. Bone marrow infiltration is seen more often in B-cell lymphomas than T-cell lymphomas
    B. Bone marrow infiltration is seen more often in high-grade B-cell lymphomas than low-grade B-cell lymphomas
    C. Paratrabecular lymphoid aggregates are almost always reactive
    D. Diffuse involvement of the bone marrow in a case of CLL imparts a favorable prognosis

30. Regarding iron stain on bone marrow aspirate slides, all of the following are true except:
    A. Normal erythroblasts have one to five iron-containing granules, distributed randomly within the cytoplasm of erythroblasts
    B. Both intracellular and extracellular iron should be assessed
    C. In healthy individuals, 20–50% of erythroblasts are sideroblasts
    D. In individuals with hemochromatosis, plasma cells in bone marrow may demonstrate hemosiderin granules

31. Lipid granulomas of the bone marrow:
    A. Are clinically significant
    B. Are typically located in paratrabecular areas
    C. Consist of fat vacuoles which are larger than marrow fat cells
    D. May have giant cells

32. Reactive or benign lymphoid aggregates may be seen in bone marrows:
    A. In states of infection
    B. In senior citizens
    C. In rheumatoid arthritis
    D. All of the above

33. Regarding reactive lymphoid aggregates in bone marrows, all are true except:
    A. They are usually few in number
    B. They are typically located in the paratrabecular areas
    C. They consist predominantly of small mature lymphocytes
    D. The lymphocytes exhibit pleomorphism

34. Bone marrow necrosis may be seen in:
    A. Sickle cell disease
    B. Acute leukemias
    C. Chronic leukemias
    D. All of the above

35. Regarding gelatinous transformation of the bone marrow:
    A. There is replacement of hematopoietic elements by fat spaces
    B. May be highlighted by Perl's stain
    C. May be seen in individuals with anorexia nervosa
    D. The peripheral blood will demonstrate leukocytosis

36. In adults, bone marrow metastasis from the following primary tumors are common except:
    A. Prostatic carcinoma
    B. Meningioma
    C. Bronchogenic carcinoma
    D. Breast cancer

37. Peripheral blood findings most characteristic of metastatic tumor to the bone marrow is:
    A. Leukoerythroblastic blood picture and presence of tear drop cells
    B. Microcytic hypochromic red cells
    C. Macrocytic anemia
    D. Leukocytosis

38. Effect of EDTA on platelets include:
    A. Decrease in MPV
    B. Increase in MPV

C. Loss of alpha granules
D. Loss of δ granules

39. Regarding reticulocytes:
    A. Normal levels in newborns are 1%
    B. Are raised in aplastic anemia
    C. Contain a network of DNA in their cytoplasm
    D. Contain ribonucleoprotein in their cytoplasm

40. Regarding the zeta potential of red cells:
    A. The zeta potential of red cells is the negative charge around red cells that prevent them from aggregating
    B. The zeta potential of red cells is the positive charge around red cells that prevent them from aggregating
    C. Agents that increase the zeta potential will result in increased ESR
    D. EDTA increases the zeta potential of red cells

Anemias: Questions 41–64

41. The following are true about reticulocytes except:
    A. They are young red cells and contain ribosomal RNA
    B. Reticulocyte count is traditionally expressed as a percentage
    C. Reticulocyte count is low in bone marrow failure patients
    D. Reticulocyte count is low in hemolytic anemia patients

42. The following are all included in the differential diagnosis of microcytic hypochromic anemia except:
    A. HbE disease
    B. β thalassemia trait
    C. Iron deficiency
    D. HbS disease

43. In a patient with β thalassemia trait, all of the following features are typically observed except:
    A. Significantly high RDW
    B. Mild microcytic hypochromic anemia
    C. Target cells on the peripheral smear
    D. Disproportionately elevated RBC count

44. In a patient with iron deficiency, which of the following features are an expected finding:
    A. Minimal anisocytosis
    B. Abundant target cells
    C. Reduced transferrin iron binding capacity
    D. Elevated levels of free erythrocyte protoporphyrin (FEP)

45. Peripheral smear and bone marrow findings in iron deficiency anemia include:
    A. Abundant target cells
    B. Thrombocytopenia
    C. Hypocellular marrow
    D. Presence of scanty, ragged vacuolated cytoplasm in the developing erythroblasts

46. Which of the following is a true statement regarding sideroblastic anemia?
    A. Sideroblastic anemia may be inherited or acquired, with the inherited form being more common
    B. In sideroblastic anemia there occurs impaired iron utilization, and excess iron is found in the Golgi apparatus
    C. Siderocytes and sideroblasts are abnormal and seen in sideroblastic anemia
    D. Acquired sideroblastic anemia may be idiopathic (primary) which is part of myelodysplastic syndrome

47. In congenital sideroblastic anemia:
    A. The red cells are most often macrocytic
    B. Is a common inherited condition
    C. In most families is transmitted as X-linked inheritance
    D. Hemoglobin electrophoresis usually demonstrates an abnormal hemoglobin

48. In lead poisoning, coarse basophilic stippling is seen and this is due to:
    A. Inhibition of the enzyme 5' pyrimidine nucleotidase
    B. Inhibition of the enzyme ferrochelatase
    C. Inhibition of the enzyme δ aminolevulinic acid dehydratase
    D. All of the above

49. Anemia of chronic disease is characterized by all of these except:
    A. Low levels of serum iron
    B. Reduced transferrin saturation
    C. Reduced iron binding capacity
    D. Reduced serum ferritin

50. Causes of macrocytic anemia include all of the following except:
    A. Acute blood loss
    B. Folate deficiency
    C. B12 deficiency
    D. Excess alcohol consumption

51. All of the following are established causes of B12 deficiency except:
    A. Diet consisting of goat milk
    B. Crohn's disease
    C. Pernicious anemia
    D. Fish tapeworm infestation

52. A 30-year-old male with long-standing history of diarrhea, has macrocytosis, Howell-Jolly bodies in RBC, target cells and small shrunken spleen. The most likely diagnosis is:
    A. Sickle cell disease
    B. Celiac disease
    C. Crohn's disease
    D. Liver disease

53. Bone marrow findings in megaloblastic anemia include all of the following except:
    A. Nuclear cytoplasmic asynchrony of developing erythroid cells
    B. Giant metamyelocytes
    C. Hypersegmented megakaryocytes
    D. Absent stainable iron in the bone marrow

54. A patient with known sickle cell disease registers with a new physician. CBC ordered by the patient's new physician demonstrates macrocytosis of the red blood cells. The most likely explanation is:
    A. Iron deficiency
    B. B12 deficiency
    C. Folate deficiency
    D. Patient is on hydroxyurea

55. In pernicious anemia, all of the following are true except:
    A. Patients may develop antiparietal cell and anti-intrinsic factor antibodies
    B. Patients are at risk of developing gastric lymphoma
    C. B12 levels are low
    D. Patients may develop neurological symptoms

56. Iron deficiency may result in the misdiagnosis of:
    A. Sickle cell trait
    B. Sickle cell disease
    C. β thalassemia trait
    D. β thalassemia disease

57. In the human body, iron is found in the largest amount in:
    A. Macrophages of the reticuloendothelial system
    B. Hemoglobin
    C. Myoglobin
    D. Enzymes

58. The total daily loss of iron in an adult male is approximately:
    A. 1 mg
    B. 2 mg
    C. 3 mg
    D. 4 mg

59. Vitamin B12
    A. Is directly required for DNA synthesis
    B. If bound to transcobalamin I is delivered to the tissues
    C. Is needed to convert methyl tetrahydrofolate (THF) to THF
    D. Is absorbed in the duodenum

60. All of the following are causes of megaloblastoid changes in the bone marrow except:
    A. B12 deficiency
    B. Hydroxyurea treatment
    C. Orotic aciduria
    D. Gout

61. In a child with anemia, bone marrow examination demonstrates erythroid hyperplasia, binuclearity and multinuclearity of the erythroid precursors. Ham's acidified serum test is positive in this patient. The most likely diagnosis is:
    A. Iron deficiency
    B. Folate deficiency

C. Congenital dyserythropoietic anemia, type I
D. Congenital dyserythropoietic anemia, type II

62. A 50-year-old male with developed macrocytic anemia (MCV is 105 fl; red cells are round and not oval). Liver function test demonstrates elevated γ glutamyl transpeptidase (GGT) as the only abnormality. Bone marrow examination shows ring sideroblasts and erythroid multinuclearity. There is vacuolation of erythroid precursors. Cytogenetics and myelodysplastic-flourescent in situ hybridization (MDS-FISH) profile are negative. The most likely diagnosis is:
    A. Myelodysplastic syndrome (MDS)
    B. Megaloblastic anemia
    C. Excess alcohol intake
    D. Hemochromatosis

63. A child with a known diagnosis of hereditary spherocytosis develops "slapped cheek" appearance as well as profound anemia. Reticulocyte response to the anemia is inadequate. A bone marrow examination is most likely to demonstrate:
    A. Hypocellular marrow with reduction of all cell lines
    B. Erythroid hyperplasia as a response to acute hemolysis
    C. Reduced erythropoiesis with giant erythroblasts and intranuclear inclusions
    D. "Owl eye " appearance, due to CMV infection in erythroid precursors

64. Characteristic feature of Fanconi's anemia include:
    A. Autosomal dominant mode of inheritance
    B. Increased risk of transformation to acute myeloid leukemia
    C. Pure red cell aplasia
    D. Skin hyperpigmentation and nail dystrophy

Hemolytic Anemias: Questions 65–84

65. All statements regarding hereditary spherocytosis is true except:
    A. May be diagnosed by flow cytometry
    B. May be diagnosed by incubated osmotic fragility test

C. When inherited, most cases are homozygous

D. The direct antiglobulin test (DAT) is typically negative

66. Regarding membrane defects of red cells, all are true except:

A. In hereditary elliptocytosis there is often defective spectrin dimer–dimer interaction.

B. In hereditary pyropoikilocytosis there is often defective spectrin dimer–dimer interaction

C. In making a diagnosis of hereditary stomatocytosis, >90% of red cells need to be stomatocytes

D. In Rh null disease, stomatocytes may be seen in the peripheral blood

67. Pyruvate kinase deficiency:

A. Is transmitted as autosomal dominant

B. Is the commonest enzyme deficiency in the TCA cycle

C. Is the commonest enzyme deficiency in the hexose monophosphate shunt

D. Can present as jaundice

68. Regarding glucose 6 phosphate dehydrogenase (G6PD) enzyme:

A. Normally two isotypes – G6PD-A and G6PD-B – can be differentiated based on electrophoretic mobility

B. The A isoform is the most common type found in all populations

C. 90% of US black men have the G6PD-A minus isoform

D. The A minus isoform has the same electrophoretic mobility as the B isoform

69. All of the following statements regarding paroxysmal nocturnal hemoglobinuria (PNH) are true except

A. PNH is transmitted as X-linked recessive

B. PNH may be diagnosed by flow cytometry

C. PNH may be diagnosed by Ham's acidified serum test

D. Occurs due to mutation of the PIG-A gene

70. Which of the following observations may be seen in a positive Ham's acidified serum test?

A. The tube with patient's red cells and patients serum, heated to 56°C shows hemolysis

B. The tube with patient's red cells and patient's serum, without addition of acid, shows hemolysis

C. The tube with patient's red cells and patient's serum, with addition of acid, show hemolysis

D. The tube with patient's red cells and patient's serum, with addition of acid and heated to 56°C shows hemolysis.

71. Regarding autoimmune hemolytic anemias:

A. In warm autoimmune hemolytic anemias (WAHA), the antibodies are often against I antigen

B. In warm autoimmune hemolytic anemia, hemolysis is typically intravascular

C. In cold hemagglutinin (CHAD) disease, antibodies are often directed against P antigen

D. Paroxysmal cold hemoglobinuria (PCH) is a rare condition and is sometimes seen in children following a viral infection.

72. Regarding the following poikilocytes, all are true except:

A. In individuals with HbSS disease, under low oxygen tension, tubular structures called tactoids deform the red cells and produce sickle cells

B. Target cells may be seen in individuals with lecithin cholesterol acyltransferase deficiency

C. Macro ovalocytes are commonly seen in individuals with hypothyroidism

D. Abundant target cells are more often seen in HbSC disease rather than in HbSS disease

73. Regarding the following poikilocytes all are true except:

A. Occasional elliptocytes may be seen in iron deficiency

B. Individuals with Rh null disease may exhibit stomatocytes in their peripheral blood

C. Echinocytes may be seen in patients with pyruvate kinase deficiency

D. Burr cells are also known as drepanocytes

74. Regarding acanthocytes

A. The word acanthocyte is derived from the Greek word for "urchin"

B. May be seen in individuals with McLeod phenotype

C. Is a feature of HbSS disease

D. These are cells with hundreds of thorny projections

75. Howell-Jolly bodies are:
A. DNA material
B. Consist of iron
C. RNA material
D. An in vitro phenomenon

76. Pyrimidine 5 nucleotidase:
A. Is an enzyme in the heme biosynthetic pathway
B. Is responsible for the degradation of RNA in red cells
C. Deficiency results in target cells
D. Deficiency results in bite cells

77. All of the following are features of parasitization of RBCs with Plasmodium falciparum except:
A. Plasmodium parasite with two chromatin dots
B. Presence of marginal forms
C. Banana- or crescent-shaped gametocytes
D. Enlarged red cells

78. In cold hemagglutinin disease (CHAD):
A. The antibody is typically IgG in nature
B. There is an association with pneumonia due to Staph aureus
C. Red cell agglutination occurs in vivo
D. Analysis of CBC values will yield low RBC count with normal hemoglobin levels

79. Established causes of microangiopathic hemolysis include all except
A. Thrombotic thrombocytopenic purpura (TTP)
B. Hemolytic uremic syndrome (HUS)
C. Disseminated intravascular coagulation (DIC)
D. Immune thrombocytopenic purpura (ITP)

80. Which of the following laboratory finding is expected in hereditary spherocytosis?
A. Increased MCHC
B. Low MCV and MCH
C. Low serum bilirubin
D. Low LDH

81. Regarding various hemolytic anemias, which statement is true:
A. Hereditary spherocytosis may be transmitted as autosomal recessive

B. G6PD deficiency may be seen in females with asymmetric lyonization
C. Myelodysplastic syndrome may result in acquired pyruvate kinase deficiency
D. All of the above

82. Which of the following tests for hereditary spherocytosis has the highest sensitivity and specificity?
A. Osmotic fragility test
B. Eosin-5-maleimide (EMA) binding test
C. Acidified glycerol lysis test (AGLT)
D. DAT

83. Regarding cryoglobulinemia:
A. HCV infection is the most common cause of type I cryoglobulinemia
B. In an individual with multiple myeloma, type III cryoglobulinemia may be seen
C. High levels of complement are expected
D. Vasculitic skin lesions may be seen

84. Gaisbock syndrome refers to:
A. Erythrocytosis seen in polycythemia rubra vera
B. Erythrocytosis seen in CML
C. Erythrocytosis seen due to dehydration
D. Erythrocytosis seen in patients with renal tumors

Hemoglobinopathies: Questions 85–109

85. An example of an embryonic hemoglobin is:
A. Hemoglobin F
B. Hemoglobin A
C. Hemoglobin A2
D. Hemoglobin Gower

86. The following are all hemoglobin adducts except:
A. HbAIII
B. HbA1c
C. HbA1d
D. Hemoglobin CS (Constant Spring)

87. Regarding hemoglobin biosynthesis:
A. The first step is formation of δ aminolevulinic acid from glycine and succinyl CoA, which takes place in the cytoplasm

B. Combination of heme with globin to form hemoglobin, in the cytoplasm

C. Conversion of protoporphyrin IX to heme by the removal of iron

D. Conversion of δ aminolevulinic acid to porphobilinogen in the mitochondria

88. Regarding hemoglobinopathies, which of the following is true:

A. There are about 100 hemoglobinopathies and most are asymptomatic

B. About 5% of the population in the world are carriers of hemoglobinopathies

C. If an individual has HbC, then their ancestry is most likely from the Carribean

D. Certain hemoglobinopathies are characterized by reduced amount of normal globin chain synthesis.

89. Which of the following is not a sickling disorder?

A. HbSS disease

B. HbSC disease

C. HbSD disease

D. HbSE disease

90. HbH disease is characterized by:

A. Deletion of one α gene

B. Deletion of two α genes

C. Deletion of three α genes

D. Deletion of four α genes

91. Regarding α thalassemia trait:

A. The condition may resemble iron deficiency

B. Individuals have significant microcytic hypochromic anemia

C. If due to alpha thalassemia 1 (-/-, α, α), which is due to cis deletion of both α genes on the same chromosome, is seen more often in the African American population

D. If due to α thalassemia 2 (-/ α, -/α), which is due to trans deletion of the α genes on two different chromosomes, is seen more often in Southeast Asian individuals

92. In α thalassemia disease:

A. Hb Bart's may be seen in the newborn

B. HbH will be evident when the patient is an adult

C. Patients have chronic hemolytic anemia

D. All of the above are true

93. An individual has microcytic hypochromic anemia (mild) with the presence of target cells on the peripheral smear. Hemoglobin electrophoresis demonstrates HbA2 (6%), HbF (3%) and HbA (91%). Iron studies are unremarkable. Patient has never received any blood transfusion. The most likely diagnosis is:

A. α thalassemia trait

B. β thalassemia trait

C. β thalassemia intermedia

D. β thalassemia major

94. An individual undergoes hemoglobin electrophoresis by the capillary method. HbA2 is detected at low levels,<1.5%. The following are possible causes:

A. α thalassemia trait

B. δ thalassemia

C. Iron deficiency

D. All of the above

95. A Greek individual undergoes hemoglobin electrophoresis for mild anemia. Results show normal HbA2 at 3.3%, HbF at 10% and the remaining hemoglobin is HbA. A possible diagnosis is:

A. β thalassemia trait

B. β thalassemia major

C. δ β thalassemia, heterozygous state

D. δ thalassemia

96. Hemoglobin S is due to a β chain defect. HbS is formed when:

A. Glutamic acid is replaced by lysine at the 26th position of the β chain

B. Glutamic acid is replaced by lysine at the 121st position of the β chain

C. Glutamic acid is replaced by lysine at the 6th position of the β chain

D. Glutamic acid is replaced by valine at the 6th position of the β chain

97. Increased levels of HbF can be seen in all of the following except:

A. HbSS disease

B. HbSS individuals on hydroxyurea

C. HbS/HPFH

D. HbAS trait

98. All of the following may be sickling disorders except:
    A. HbAS trait
    B. HbS/β zero thalassemia
    C. HbSS disease
    D. HbS/HPFH

99. A clinically important abnormal hemoglobin which is typically underproduced and thus present in low quantities is:
    A. HbD-Punjab
    B. HbE
    C. Hb Lepore
    D. HbD-Los Angeles

100. Physiological causes of elevated levels of HbF include:
    A. Advanced age
    B. Aplastic anemia
    C. Pregnancy
    D. Puberty

101. Examples of clinically significant fast hemoglobin on agarose gel electrophoresis is:
    A. HbJ
    B. HbI
    C. HbN
    D. Hb Bart's

102. In an individual who has been diagnosed with Hb S/Hb G disease, which of the following hemoglobins may be seen:
    A. HbA
    B. HbG
    C. HbS/G
    D. All of the above

103. Which of the following methodologies for the analysis of hemoglobins have the highest incidence of carryover from one sample to the next?
    A. HPLC
    B. Gel electrophoresis
    C. Capillary electrophoresis
    D. None of the above

104. A known individual with HbSS disease undergoes red cell exchange. Posthemoglobin electrophoresis shows HbA 80%, HbS 12%, HbF 4% and HbC 4%. The most likely explanation for the presence of HbC is:
    A. Spontaneous new mutation
    B. Previous diagnosis of HbSS was wrong and the patient actually has HbSC disease
    C. One of the RBCs that was used for transfusion was from a HbAC (C trait) donor
    D. Carryover from the previous sample that was tested

105. Regarding methemoglobinemia:
    A. May be due to hemoglobin variants such as HbM
    B. In normal individuals, methemoglobin levels are less than 10%
    C. With methemoglobinemia the color of the blood remains bright red
    D. The iron in methemoglobin is in the ferrous state (Fe2+)

106. An adult with sickle cell disease exhibits target cells and Howell-Jolly bodies in his peripheral smear. The most likely explanation for these findings is:
    A. Significant hemolysis
    B. Autosplenectomy
    C. Chronic hepatitis B infection
    D. Folate deficiency

107. Which of the following statements regarding methemoglobin (Hi) is false?
    A. Methemoglobin (Hi) is hemoglobin where the iron is in the ferric state (Fe+++)
    B. Hi has increased affinity to bind with oxygen
    C. Causes of elevated Hi include hereditary and acquired causes
    D. With elevated levels of Hi, cyanosis is an expected finding

108. Risk of developing renal medullary carcinoma is higher in:
    A. HbSS disease
    B. HbAS trait
    C. HbSC disease
    D. All of the above

109. Regarding abnormal hemoglobins:
    A. High oxygen affinity hemoglobin such as Hb Chesapeake will result in a leftward shift of the oxygen dissociation curve
    B. Low oxygen affinity hemoglobin such as Hb Beth Israel will result in a rightward shift of the oxygen dissociation curve
    C. Unstable hemoglobin such as Hb Hasharon will result in the precipitation of the abnormal hemoglobin if lysed red cells are incubated with 17% isopropanol
    D. All of the above are true

Answers to Chapter 1

1. C	29. A	57. B	85. D
2. B	30. B	58. A	86. D
3. A	31. D	59. C	87. B
4. C	32. D	60. D	88. B
5. D	33. B	61. D	89. D
6. A	34. D	62. C	90. C
7. D	35. C	63. C	91. A
8. D	36. B	64. B	92. D
9. C	37. A	65. C	93. B
10. C	38. B	66. C	94. D
11. D	39. D	67. D	95. C
12. A	40. B	68. A	96. D
13. C	41. D	69. A	97. D
14. B	42. D	70. C	98. A
15. C	43. A	71. D	99. C
16. D	44. D	72. C	100. C
17. A	45. D	73. D	101. D
18. D	46. D	74. B	102. D
19. B	47. C	75. A	103. A
20. D	48. A	76. B	104. C
21. A	49. D	77. D	105. A
22. C	50. A	78. D	106. B
23. D	51. A	79. D	107. B
24. D	52. B	80. A	108. D
25. D	53. D	81. D	109. D
26. B	54. D	82. B	
27. C	55. B	83. D	
28. C	56. C	84. C	

Answers to Chapter 1 (with Explanations)

1. C

Erythropoiesis involves maturation of erythroblasts to red cells. The stages in between include basophilic normoblast (early normoblast), polychromatic normoblast (intermediate normoblast), orthochromatic normoblast (late normoblast) and reticulocyte. The erythropoietic elements are typically seen as clusters (or islands) surrounding macrophages. The macrophages provide nutrition to the developing and to the maturing cells and are referred to as nurse cells. They also phagocytize defective erythropoietic precursors. Erythropoiesis occurs close to sinusoids, not in the paratrabecular areas. Proerythroblasts are large cells with deep blue cytoplasm and a large nucleus. A Golgi hof may be apparent. The nuclei have nucleoli. Nucleoli are not apparent in subsequent cells. The nuclei of the normoblasts become more and more clumped and in late normoblasts the nuclei are dark and pyknotic. The cytoplasm of the normoblasts changes from blue (in early normoblasts) to bluish grey (in intermediate normoblasts) to orange-pink tinge (in late normoblasts). These changes denote increased amount of hemoglobin in the cytoplasm. Once the nucleus is extruded the cell is known as a reticulocyte, which is converted to a mature red cell in approximately three days.

2. B

CD 71 is the transferrin receptor and is present in erythroid precursors. It is not present in mature red cells. CD34 is an immature marker and not confined to erythroid precursors. It is thus present in myeloblasts and lymphoblasts. CD41 is platelet glycoprotein IIb and CD61 is platelet glycoprotein IIIa.

3. A

Heme biosynthesis starts with the formation of δ aminolevulinic acid from glycine and succinyl CoA, which is the rate-limiting step. This takes place in the mitochondrion. The next few steps of heme biosynthesis takes place in the cytoplasm. The last step, which is the formation of heme from protoporphyrin IX (addition of Fe with the help of the enzyme ferrochelatase), again takes place in the mitochondrion. Heme then moves to the cytoplasm and combines with the globin chains to form hemoglobin. When there is iron deficiency, then the enzyme ferrochelatase substitutes zinc in place of iron. Zinc protoporphyrin is thus formed. In iron deficiency, levels of zinc protoporphyrin are increased.

4. C

Primary granules are seen in abundance at the promyelocyte stage. They are reddish-purple. The promyelocytes of the three granulocytes cannot be differentiated by light microscopy. Myelocytes have secondary granules, also known as specific granules. The three different granulocytes can be differentiated from this stage. Blasts and promyelocytes have nucleoli. Myelocytes, metamyelocytes, bands and mature granulocytes do not have nucleoli. Blasts, promyelocytes and myelocytes are all capable of cell division. Metamyelocytes and more mature cells are not. Granulopoiesis in a normal marrow takes place in the paratrabecular region as well close to arterioles.

5. D

The normal sequence of maturation for erythropoiesis is proerythroblast to basophilic normoblast to polychromatic normoblast to orthochromatic normoblast to reticulocyte to a mature red cell. The proerythroblasts is the largest cell. Proerythroblasts have nucleoli. Subsequently nucleoli are absent. Erythropoiesis typically occurs in islands close to sinusoids.

6. A

Megakaryocytes mature through endomitosis, where nuclear DNA content increases in multiples of two. However, there is no cytoplasmic or nuclear division. Normal development of megakaryocytes is regulated by multiple cytokines and one principal one is thrombopoietin. Megakaryocytes can be seen to go through three stages of maturation, stages I, II and III. In stage I, the megakaryocytes have strong basophilic cytoplasm and high nuclear cytoplasmic ratio. In stage II the cytoplasm is less basophilic and has some granules. The N:C ratio is lower. In the third and final stage, which denotes mature megakaryocytes, the cytoplasm is abundant with granules. The margin of the cytoplasm is, however, agranular. The cytoplasm is weakly basophilic. Hematopoietic cells may be seen within the cytoplasm of megakaryocytes. The cells are not destroyed. This is referred to as emperipolesis. Clustering of more than three megakaryocytes is considered to be abnormal. They may be seen in myelodysplasia as well as regenerating marrows.

7. D

Osteoblasts and therefore osteocytes are derived from mesenchymal origin. Chondrocytes are also mesenchymal in origin. In contrast, osteoclasts are derived from hematopoietic stem cells. They are formed from the fusion of monocytic cells.

8. D

Erythroblasts are found as distinctive islands and surround a macrophage. The cells closest to the macrophages are less mature than those which are distant. The macrophage has cytoplasmic processes which envelop erythroblasts. These macrophages are known as "nurse" cells. The macrophages can engulf defective erythroblasts. Erythropoiesis occurs close to the sinusoids. With Giemsa stain the erythroblasts are deeply basophilic with a small golgi hof. Artifactual shrinking of the cytoplasm is seen in paraffin-embedded sections. This does not occur with plastic-embedded sections.

9. C

Myeloblasts are found in the paratrabecular areas as well as close to arterioles. At the metamyelocyte stage they are found close to sinusoids, and at the PMN stage they can cross the wall of sinusoids and enter into the circulation. Myeloblasts, promyelocytes and myelocytes are capable of cell division. It is from the myelocyte stage that cells of the three granulocytic lineages can be discerned. This is due to the nature of the granules. Indented myeloid precursors are known as metamyelocytes.

10. C

Megakaryocytes are found close to sinusoids. Paratrabecular location of megakaryocytes is considered abnormal. Megakaryocytes as they mature undergo DNA replication without nuclear division (endomitosis/endoreduplication). In a normal marrow, megakaryocytes may range from 4N to 32N. The nucleus is large and lobulated. As megakaryocytes mature, the cytoplasm appears less basophilic and has azurophilic granules. On the basis of maturity, megakaryocytes may be divided into three groups. Group I cells are most immature and group III cells are fully mature. Group III cells do not synthesize DNA. Megakaryocytes may engulf hematopoietic cells. They are actually within the membrane system within the megakaryocytes. They are not destroyed. This process is called emperipolesis. Clusters of megakaryocytes greater than three is considered to be abnormal.

11. D

IL- is the key cytokine for eosinophils. IL-3 and GM-CSF are additional agents.

12. A

Neutrophils have two types of granules. Primary granules are also known as azurophilic granules and contain lysosomal enzymes and peroxidase (hence the name MPO). They are found in immature granulocytic cells. Secondary or specific granules are found in mature cells and contain lactoferrin (which binds with iron).

13. C

On average, each proerythroblast forms eight reticulocytes. The average transit time for this is approximately five days. In acute anemia this transit time is short. It can be as little as one to two days. These red cells may be macrocytic and bear i antigen in contrast to the I antigen. They may also increase HbF concentration. Stress erythropoiesis is also associated with Pappenheimer bodies, basophilic stippling and Howell-Jolly bodies.

14. B

Megakaryocytes are approximately 0.05%–0.1% of hematopoietic cells in a normal bone marrow. Each megakaryocyte gives rise to 1,000–3,000 platelets. Megakaryocytes are polyploidy and contain 2N–64N of DNA. The mean value is 16N in humans. Immature megakaryocytes have little basophilic cytoplasm. As megakaryocytes mature, cytoplasm becomes abundant and appears violet in color.

15. C

When compared to adult CBC values, normal values for neonates and children differ considerably with the exception of platelet count. The normal platelet count for all ages ranges from 150,000/uL to 350,000/uL. One easy way to remember is that in general neonates have all counts higher (e.g. hemoglobin, RBC count, WBC count) and cells are in general bigger (e.g. MCV).

The normal hemoglobin level in neonates ranges from 16 to 20 gm/dl. This then declines to 9–11 gm/dl at around 3–6 months. By adolescent stage adult values are reached.

16. D

For hemoglobin measurement the spectrophotometric method is used. At first the red cells are lysed. The ferrous ion of hemoglobin is oxidized by potassium ferrocyanide to the ferric form. Potassium cyanide converts the ferric form to stable cyanmethemoglobin. However, sulfhemoglobin is not converted to cyanmethhemoglobin. Other reagents are used to lower the pH and accelerate the reaction as well as to reduce turbidity. Absorbance of light at 540 nm is measured. Smokers have higher than normal levels of carboxyhemoglobin. Carboxyhemoglobin absorbs more light at 540 nm. Thus smokers have higher values of hemoglobin.

17. A

In oxyhemoglobin, iron is in the ferrous state. In methemoglobin, iron is in the ferric state.

18. D

Leukocytosis, paraproteinemia and hyperlipidemia are important causes of falsely elevated hemoglobin levels.

19. B

For the RBC indices, the following equations are important:

Hct= MCV X RBC count
MCH=Hb/RBC count
MCHC=Hb/Hct

Using the RBC histogram a perpendicular line is drawn from the peak to the X axis. The point where this line cuts the X axis is the MCV of the RBCs. RDW, a measure of the variation of size of RBCs (i.e. anisocytosis), is also done from the RBC histogram.

20. D

In cold hemagglutinin disease (CHAD), clumped red cells may be counted as single RBCs. The RBC count is thus falsely low. The Hct is also low. The hemoglobin level is accurate as red cells are lysed prior to hemoglobin estimation. MCHC in CHAD is high (MCHC=Hb/Hct). Thus, abnormally high MCHC is a tip off for CHAD. If the blood is warmed and CBC analysis is repeated, correct values will now be obtained. MCHC values are also increased in hereditary spherocytosis and in patients with hemoglobin variants such as sickle cell disease and hemoglobin C disease.

21. A

Nucleated RBCs can be counted as lymphocytes, thus spuriously elevating the WBC. However, when the WBC count is performed in the "NRBC" mode, the nucleated red cells are lysed and an accurate WBC count results.

22. C

When blood is collected with EDTA as the anticoagulant, there may occur platelet clumps as well as platelet satellitism. In platelet satellitism, platelets bind with ligands on neutrophils and thus are excluded from counting. Traumatic venepuncture with activation of clotting is another cause of thrombocytopenia. If there is a significant number of large platelets, then these large platelets are falsely counted as RBCs rather than platelets, resulting in a lower than true platelet count. Fragmented RBCs may be falsely counted as platelets, thus increasing the platelet count.

23. D

Wright-Giemsa stains paraproteins blue. Thus, when there is a significant amount of paraprotein, peripheral smear slides may appear blue to the naked eye.

24. D

All of the above conditions will demonstrate increased promyelocytes with paucity of more mature cells. However, promyelocytes seen in APL will demonstrate Auer rods with no Golgi hof. Immunophenotype of abnormal promyelocytes seen in APL will also be different.

25. D

Established causes of bone marrow granulomas include infections, sarcoidosis, malignancies, and drugs. Examples of infections include Tuberculosis, fungal infections and brucellosis. Examples of malignancies include Hodgkin and non-Hodgkin lymphomas and metastatic diseases. Lipogranulomas may also be seen in bone marrows. These are focal aggregates of macrophages with lipid vacuoles. Lymphocytes, plasma cells and eosinophils are seen associated with them. They are benign in nature.

26. B

Gaucher's disease is due to the lack of the enzyme glucocerebrocidase. The cytoplasm of the macrophages have a wrinkled tissue paper appearance. The macrophages are also periodic acid-Schiff (PAS) positive. Very similar to Gaucher cells are pseudo Gaucher cells. These cells are macrophages with similar appearance of their cytoplasm. They are seen in conditions with high cell membrane turnover. Examples include CML, hemoglobinopathies and myeloma. Infections with mycobacterium avium intracellulare (MAI) with acid fast bacilli stain may also mimic Gaucher cells. In Niemann-Pick disease there occurs deficiency of the enzyme sphingomyelinase. Here we see foamy macrophages with bubbly cytoplasm.

27. C

Sea blue histiocytes are again macrophages that contain ceroid. They appear blue-green with Giemsa stain. They are PAS positive. With H&E stain the cytoplasm of the macrophages appear yellow-brown. They are usually seen in conditions with high cell turnover such as CML, sickle cell disease.

28. C

One of the most common causes of a dry tap is faulty technique by the person performing the procedure. However, in certain hematologic conditions it should not be surprising to fail to obtain an aspirate. Such conditions include aplastic anemia, packed marrow (esp. acute leukemias), and bone marrow fibrosis. Hairy cell leukemia is a distinct entity which is typically associated with a dry tap.

29. A

Bone marrow infiltrates are actually seen more often in B-cell lymphomas than in T-cell lymphomas. They are seen more often in low-grade B-cell lymphomas than in high-grade B-cell lymphomas. The various patterns of lymphoid infiltrates include nodular (this type may be paratrabecular and non-paratrabecular), interstitial (neoplastic cells are seen among the hematopoietic cells), intrasinusoidal, focal and diffuse. Paratrabecular lymphoid aggregates are a classical feature of follicular lymphoma involving the bone marrow. Diffuse lymphoid involvement imparts a poor prognosis.

30. B

In a bone marrow aspirate slide that is stained for iron, there will be both intracellular and extracellular iron. The extracellular iron is derived from crushed macrophages. Iron stains are prone to artifactual deposits and it is difficult to distinguish from these artifactual deposits and extracellular iron. Thus, it is best only to assess intracellular iron. Normal erythroblasts have 1–5 iron-containing granules, distributed randomly within the cytoplasm of erythroblasts. In healthy individuals, 20–50% of erythroblasts are sideroblasts. Abnormal sideroblasts include those in which iron granules are increased in number or increased in size or distributed in a ring manner (ring sideroblasts). In certain conditions such as chronic alcoholism and hemochromatosis, plasma cells may contain hemosiderin granules.

31. D

Lipid granulomas of the bone marrow are sometimes seen in up to 9% of bone marrows examined. They consist of fat vacuoles which vary in size but are smaller than marrow fat cells. The fat vacuoles may be located within macrophages or in extracellular spaces. They are typically located near sinusoids or lymphoid aggregates. They may have lymphocytes, plasma cells, eosinophils or even giant cells. Lipid granulomas are of no clinical significance.

32. D

Reactive lymphoid aggregates may be seen in a variety of conditions. These include infection, inflammation, hemolytic states, autoimmune conditions and with increasing age.

33. B

Reactive lymphoid aggregates are usually few in number. The aggregates consist predominantly of small mature lymphocytes which exhibit pleomorphism. In addition to lymphocytes there may be some plasma cells, macrophages and even mast cells, immunoblasts and eosinophils. They are rarely located in the paratrabecular area. They are most often seen close to small blood vessels.

34. D

Bone marrow necrosis may be seen in a wide variety of conditions. These include sickle cell disease, leukemias, lymphomas, metastatic disease of the bone marrow, Caisson disease and antiphospholipid syndrome. Extensive necrosis may result in pancytopenia. There may be recovery of hematopoietic elements as well as bone. There may be fibrosis, which at times may be extensive.

35. C

Gelatinous transformation of bone marrow is also known as serous atrophy or serous degeneration. Here there is loss of hematopoietic cells as well as loss of fat cells. This loss is replaced by ground substance. In the aspirate slide there is increased amorphous material which may be granular or fibrillary. In the biopsy slide, the amorphous material typically is pale pink material. Gelatinous transformation may be seen in anorexia nervosa, cachexia, chronic debilitating conditions, AIDS and at sites exposed to high-dose radiation.

36. B

In adults, prostate cancer, lung and breast cancer are common causes of metastasis to the bone marrow. In children, neuroblastoma, rhabdomyosarcoma, retinoblastoma and PNETs are tumors that may metastasize to the bone marrow.

37. A

The most characteristic peripheral blood finding, when the bone marrow is involved with a metastatic tumor, is presence of nucleated red cells as well as left shift in the WBC series with presence of blasts. This is referred to as leukoerythroblastic blood picture. In addition, there may be tear drop red cells. These features may be seen in any condition where there is bone marrow infiltration (e.g.

by fibrous tissue). Anemia due to bone marrow infiltration is referred to as myelopthisic anemia.

38. B

EDTA increases MPV. This is due to shape change in the platelets where they become spherical from their discoid shape.

39. D

Normal levels of reticulocytes in newborns are 5–7%, falling quickly to adult levels (1%) at the end of the first week of life. They contain ribonucleoprotein, which can be stained with supravital dyes such as new methylene blue and brilliant cresyl blue. Reticulocytes remain in the circulation for 2–3 days before becoming mature red cells.

40. B

Red cells have sialic acid residues on their surface. Presence of these residues result in a negative charge on the surface of red cells. Positively charged ions in the plasma surround the surface of the red cells. This is the zeta potential. The zeta potential helps red cells from aggregating. Any agent that reduces the zeta potential will result in increased aggregation of red cells. Thus ESR will be increased. EDTA does not affect the zeta potential. Heparin does. Thus, blood collected in heparin is not suitable for ESR testing.

41. D

Reticulocytes are young red cells that have been recently released from the bone marrow. They contain ribosomal RNA. Supravital staining such as brilliant cresyl blue precipitates the ribosomes and a reticular network is apparent. Reticulocytes can be subdivided into four groups. Group I reticulocytes have most amount of reticulum and appear as a large clump on staining with a supravital stain. In group IV, a few granules are evident. Increased reticulocytes is referred to as polychromasia. Reticulocytes are traditionally expressed as a percentage of RBCs. It is more meaningful to use an alternative method of expression, for example, the corrected reticulocyte count. This is calculated as follows:

Corrected Reticulocyte count= reticulocyte percentage X patient Hct/ normal Hct

In situations where the bone marrow is not able to produce adequate red cells the reticulocyte count will be low. Examples include aplastic anemia and acute leukemias. In hemolytic anemias the bone marrow compensates by increased erythropoiesis, and increased reticulocyte counts are observed.

42. D

Causes of microcytic hypochromic anemia include iron deficiency, anemia of chronic disease, thalassemias and hemoglobinopathies. A notable exception is HbS.

43. A

The RDW is a useful discriminator between iron deficiency and β thalassemia trait in a case of microcytic hypochromic anemia. In iron deficiency it is significantly elevated. In β thalassemia trait it is normal or very mildly elevated. In fact anisocytosis in iron deficiency is seen before development of microcytic hypochromic red cells. In β thalassemia trait the hemoglobin may be normal or the patient may be mildly anemic. Target cells are usually seen; in some they may be infrequent or even absent.

44. D

Iron deficiency results in microcytic hypochromic anemia, with significant anisocytosis. Actually anisocytosis precedes development of microcytic hypochromic red cells. Occasional pencil cells and occasional or rare target cells are seen. Presence of abundant target cells should prompt search for other explanations. Patients with iron deficiency may also at times exhibit thrombocytosis. Iron studies should demonstrate low serum iron, low serum ferritin and low serum transferrin saturation. Please note ferritin is an acute phase reactant. Levels may be raised in inflammatory states and cause confusion. Serum transferrin iron binding capacity is increased. When there is inadequate iron, excess protoporphyrin which was destined to form heme accumulates within red cells. Elevated levels of FEP can also be seen in situations where iron utilization is blocked such as in anemia of chronic disease, lead poisoning and sideroblastic anemia. With iron deficiency there is increased production of transferrin receptor. Transferrin receptors are found in the cell membrane. A truncated form of the receptor is found in the soluble form in the serum. Increased levels of transferrin receptors are also seen with increased erythropoiesis or ineffective erythropoiesis.

Patients with β thalassemia trait also have microcytic hypochromic red cells with minimal anisocytosis. The RBC count is disproportionately elevated when compared to the hemoglobin level. Target cells are found in increased numbers (much more than seen with iron deficiency).

Individuals with anemia of chronic disease have decreased serum iron, decreased transferrin saturation. However, serum transferrin iron binding capacity is decreased. FEP is raised but soluble serum transferrin receptor levels are normal. Red cells are either normocytic normochromic or microcytic hypochromic.

45. D

Iron deficiency anemia is characterized by microcytic hypochromic red cells with anisocytosis, pencil-(or cigar)shaped red cells and occasional target cells. Abundant target cells are not a feature of iron deficiency. Abundant target cells may be seen in liver disease or hemoglobinopathies. The platelet count is normal or raised. This is especially true if the patient is bleeding. The bone marrow is usually of normal cellularity. Sometimes there is erythroid hyperplasia. The developing erythroblasts exhibit scanty, ragged vacuolated cytoplasm. There is significantly reduced/absent bone marrow stainable iron.

46. D

Sideroblastic anemia is due to abnormal iron metabolism, where iron cannot be utilized and is sequestered in mitochondria. The mitochondria in immature erythroid precursors are distributed in a ring manner around the nucleus. Iron stains will demonstrate presence of iron in a ring distribution. These cells are referred to as ringed sideroblasts. Presence of ringed sideroblasts are abnormal. Siderocyte is any red cell with iron. Sideroblasts are immature erythroid precursors with iron. Both are physiological. Sideroblastic anemia may be inherited or acquired. Inherited forms are rare. The acquired form may be primary (part of MDS) or secondary due to drugs (e.g. antituberculous drugs), lead or alcohol. In sideroblastic anemia serum iron is increased, TIBC is decreased or normal, transferrin saturation is increased. Ferritin levels are high.

47. C

Sideroblastic anemia may be congenital or acquired. There are several forms of congenital sideroblastic anemia. These are X-linked sideroblastic anemia due to mutation of the 5-aminolevulinic acid synthase gene(ALAS2) or mutation in the ABC gene, autosomal recessive sideroblastic anemia, mitochondrial DNA defect and as part of Wolfram syndrome (diabetes insipidus, diabetes mellitus, optic atrophy and deafness in association with sideroblastic or megaloblastic anemia).

The X-linked sideroblastic anemia is the most common type of congenital sideroblastic anemia.

48. A

Lead poisoning causes inhibition of all of the above enzymes. Inhibition of δ aminolevulinic acid dehydratase prevents the formation of porphobilinogen. Levels of δ aminolevulinic acid accumulates. Such elevations are also seen in acute intermittent porphyria. Inhibition of ferrochelatase results in inhibition of iron combining with protoporphyrin IX to form heme. Free protoporphyrin IX then forms a metal chelate with zinc. This results in elevated levels of zinc protoporphyrin. 5' pyrimidine nucleotidase is responsible for the degradation of RNA material within reticulocytes. Undegraded RNA material results in basophilic stippling.

49. D

Anemia of chronic disease is a disorder seen in states of chronic infection or inflammation or less often in malignancy. It is thought that cytokines that are released from inflammatory cells cause inadequate release of iron from reticuloendothelial cells for erythropoiesis. Bone marrow iron stores are adequate. There is inadequate response to erythropoietin as well as reduced RBC survival. Anemia of chronic disease may manifest as normocytic normochromic, as well as microcytic hypochromic anemia. The reticulocyte count is reduced.

See Table 1.1 to contrast iron deficiency, anemia of chronic disease, and thalassemia trait.

50. A

Causes of macrocytic anemia include folate/B12 deficiency, alcohol, hypothyroidism, chronic liver disease and pregnancy. Macrocytic anemia can be megaloblastic macrocytic or normoblastic macrocytic. In megaloblastic macrocytic anemia the erythroid precursors are large and macrocytosis in the peripheral blood is marked, classically the MCV is >120fl. Causes include folate and B12 deficiency. In normoblastic macrocytic anemia the erythroid precursors are not large and macrocytosis in the peripheral blood is not as marked, classically <120fl. Causes include alcohol, chronic liver disease, hypothyroidism, and pregnancy. In megaloblastic macrocytic anemia the red cells are oval in shape. They are referred to as oval macrocytes. Hypersegmented PMNs (PMNS with >5 segments) may be seen. The bone marrow exhibits erythroid hyperplasia with large erythroid precursors. Large granulocytic precursors are also observed. There may be morphologic evidence of dysplasia. Megaloblastic anemia may also produce cytopenias including pancytopenia. Thus, features may mimic myelodysplasia.

51. A

VITAMIN B12 is absent from plant sources. B12 absorption requires presence of intrinsic factor released by parietal cells of the stomach. The site of B12 absorption is the terminal ileum. Once absorbed, transcobalamin I and II serve as carriers. It is transcobalamin II which delivers vitamin B12 to tissues.

Table 1.1

	Iron deficiency anemia	Anemia of chronic disease	Thalassemia trait
Serum iron	Reduced	Reduced	Normal
Serum ferritin	Reduced	Normal or increased	Normal
Transferrin saturation	Reduced	Reduced	Normal
Transferrin iron binding capacity	Increased	Reduced or normal; not increased	Normal
Zinc protoporphyrin	Increased	Increased	Normal or increased
Soluble transferrin receptor	Increased	Reduced or normal	Increased
Bone marrow iron store	Reduced	Not reduced; often increased	Present

Thus, vegans have no dietary intake of B12. Gastrectomy or pernicious anemia (autoimmune destruction of gastric mucosa) will also result in B12 deficiency. Crohn's disease (which affects the terminal ileum) or ileal resection and transcobalamin II deficiency will also result in B12 deficiency. Bacterial colonization of the small intestine, fish tapeworm infestation, and Imerslund-Grasbeck syndrome (congenital specific malabsorption) are some unusual causes of B12 deficiency.

Diet consisting of goat milk results in folate deficiency.

52. B

Howell-Jolly bodies, target cells and acanthocytes are features of hyposplenism. Hyposplenism without history of removal of spleen can be seen in sickle cell disease and celiac disease. Celiac disease is associated with bowel motion disturbance. Thus, the unifying diagnosis is celiac disease with splenic atrophy. The mechanism of hyposplenism in celiac disease is not completely understood.

53. D

In megaloblastic anemia cytoplasmic maturation characterized by hemoglobinization takes place. However, the nuclei are abnormally retained an open and lacy. This is nuclear cytoplasmic asynchrony. This feature may also be seen in myelodysplasia. Other erythroid features include nuclear bridging and multinucleation. Erythroid and granulocytic precursors may be large. Megakaryocytes may demonstrate abnormal open chromatin pattern with hypersegmentation. In patients with megaloblastic anemia without iron deficiency there is usually excessive iron granulation of erythroblasts.

54. D

Patients with sickle cell disease are often given hydroxyurea. This increases the relative percentage of HbF with reduction in the relative percentage of HbS. Thus, the likelihood of various sickle cell crises are reduced. Hydroxyurea is, however, antifolate. Thus patients develop macrocytosis. This phenomenon is useful for monitoring compliance of patients who are prescribed hydroxyurea.

55. B

Pernicious anemia is an autoimmune disorder. Patient may develop antiparietal cell (90%

of patients) and anti-intrinsic factor (50% of patients) antibodies. Anti-intrinsic factor antibody is considered to be more specific for the condition. Patients also develop gastric atrophy and are predisposed to gastric carcinoma not lymphoma. Pernicious anemia like other autoimmune disorders are associated with presence of other autoimmune conditions. B12 levels are low and individuals with very low B12 levels may develop neurological features such as peripheral neuropathy and subacute combined degeneration of the spinal cord.

56. C.

Iron deficiency causes levels of HbA2 to be falsely low. β thalassemia trait by hemoglobin electrophoresis will demonstrate HbA2 levels greater than 3.5%. With concomitant iron deficiency, hemoglobin A2 levels may be less than 3.5%, thereby missing the opportunity for diagnosing β thalassemia trait.

57. B

The majority of the iron (about 60–65%) in the human body is found in hemoglobin. Typically there is 500 mg for every liter of blood. The second largest store of iron is in the macrophages of the reticuloendothelial system. Iron in myoglobin and some enzymes contribute toward a smaller portion of the total body iron.

58. A

The total daily loss of iron in an adult male and postmenopausal female is approximately 1mg. Thus, total daily requirement is 1mg. However, approximately 10% of ingested iron is absorbed. Thus the required dietary intake for adult males and postmenopausal females is 10mg. The requirement for menstruating females is higher and for pregnant women the requirement is even higher.

59. C

Vitamin B12 at first binds to R binder in the stomach. Pancreatic enzymes separate B12 from the R binder protein and then B12 binds to Intrinsic factor. B12 is absorbed in the terminal ileum and binds to transcobalamin (TC) II. In the peripheral blood B12 is also bound to TC I (derived from granulocytes and monocytes). This accounts for the majority of B12 in peripheral blood. However, TC I does not deliver B12 to the tissues. Also, in inflammatory states when there is high levels of inflammatory cells, TC I levels are high. B12 levels are also high in such situations.

Vitamin B12 is not directly required for DNA synthesis. It is required to convert methyl THF to THF. THF is required for DNA synthesis.

60. D

Megaloblastic anemia may be due to folate deficiency, B12 deficiency, anti-metabolite therapy (e.g. hydroxyurea, methotrexate), orotic aciduria, and/or erythroleukemia.

61. D

Congenital dyserythropoietic anemias (CDA) are inherited conditions, manifesting as anemias at an early age. Other features include splenomegaly, jaundice and gallstones (due to ineffective erythropoiesis and shortened RBC life span). There are three types (I, II and III) of which type II is the most common and is transmitted as autosomal recessive (type I is also transmitted as autosomal recessive and type III is transmitted as autosomal dominant). The peripheral blood displays anisocytosis and poikilocytosis (e.g. fragmented red cells). Reticulocyte response to the anemia is inadequate. Basophilic stippling is usually present. Bone marrow examination shows erythroid hyperplasia with features of dyserythropoiesis. Binuclearity and multinuclearity are seen. In CDA types I and III megaloblastic features are seen. In type II erythropoiesis is typically normoblastic. Nuclear karyorrhexis is seen in all types. In type II Ham's acidified serum test is positive. This type is also known as hereditary erythroblastic multinuclearity with positive acidified serum lysis test (HEMPAS).

62. C

Isolated level of increased GGT is seen with excessive alcohol intake. Alcohol is a well established hematologic toxin. The peripheral blood demonstrates macrocytosis. The macrocytosis is not as marked as seen in megaloblastic anemia (where MCV is may be 120fl or higher). Oval macrocytes and hypersegmented PMNs are not seen. Target cells may be seen. Heavy alcohol intake and acute liver damage may result in Zieve's syndrome. Here there is hemolytic anemia with hyperlipidemia. Spherocytes and irregularly contracted cells are seen in the peripheral blood. Alcohol is also associated with increased iron stores. Bone marrow may have ring sideroblasts. Dyserythropoiesis is seen. Erythroid as well as granulocytic precursors may exhibit features of vacuolation. A misdiagnosis of MDS is possible.

63. C

Parvovirus B19 may induce aplastic crisis in individuals with a background of chronic hemolysis. It may also produce "slapped cheek" appearance in infected individuals. The infection is transient in immunocompetent individuals. In immunocompromised patients clinical effect may be sustained. There is reduced erythropoiesis with giant erythroblasts and intranuclear inclusions. Immunostains may be used for confirmation.

64. B

Fanconi's anemia is the commonest cause of constitutional aplastic anemias. It is transmitted as autosomal recessive and results from defective DNA repair. Aplastic anemia develops by mid childhood and subsequently there is increased risk of progression to AML. Developmental defects such as short stature, renal defects and mental retardation are additional features. Dyskeratosis congenita is another, although rare cause of consituitional bone marrow aplasia. It is characterized by skin hyperpigmentation and nail dystrophy. Shwachman-Diamond syndrome is a rare genetic disorder with aplastic anemia, which may progress to myelodysplasia and AML. In addition, patients may also have exocrine pancreatic dysfunction and resultant growth failure. Diamond-Blackfan anemia is a condition with pure red cell aplasia. It is also constitutional.

65. C

Hereditary spherocytosis is the most common cause of hereditary hemolytic anemia in individuals of northern European descent. It is transmitted as autosomal dominant. However, in about 20–25% of cases it occurs due to spontaneous mutation. Most inherited cases are due to heterozygous states. Homozygous states are usually lethal. In hereditary spherocytosis there occurs abnormalities of red cell membrane proteins. There may be deficiency of spectrin, deficiency of spectrin and ankyrin (combined), band 3 deficiency or protein 4.1 defects.

The spherocytes are cells without central pallor. These cells are destroyed prematurely by the spleen. Diagnosis includes osmotic fragility test. In 10–20% of cases, this test may be negative. Incubated osmotic fragility test may be helpful. Flow cytometry is also available for diagnosis of hereditary spherocytosis.

66. C

Hereditary elliptocytosis may be diagnosed when >20% of red cells are elliptocytes. This condition is transmitted as autosomal dominant. There are three forms of the condition: the common form, the spherocytic form and the stomatocytic form. In this condition the RBC cytoskeleton is disrupted. The most frequent defect is spectrin dimer–dimer interaction. Hereditary pyropoikilocytosis is also thought to be due to defect in spectrin dimer–dimer interaction. The peripheral smear demonstrates striking anisocytosis and poikilocytosis. RBC fragments and microspherocytes are seen in abundance. Hereditary pyropoikilocytosis is typically a severe form of congenital hemolytic anemia. In contrast, hereditary elliptocytosis may range from asymptomatic carrier state to a severe hemolytic form.

Unlike hereditary spherocytosis, hereditary elliptocytosis and hereditary pyropoikilocytosis, hereditary stomatocytosis is not due to an inherited defect of the RBC membrane cytoskeleton. Rather it is due to abnormal RBC membrane cation permeability. It is also transmitted as autosomal dominant. >35% of red cells with stomatocytic form is usually enough to make the diagnosis.

Rh null disease is when an individual lacks all Rh determinants. This condition is associated with stomatocytes and spherocytes in their peripheral blood.

67. D

In red cells, glucose is utilized through the glycolytic pathway or the hexose monophosphate shunt (also known as the pentose phosphate pathway). Glycolysis generates ATP which is required to maintain the sodium/potassium ATPase pump. This pump ensures extrusion of sodium and water from the RBC and thus helps to maintain the biconcave shape. The hexose monophosphate shunt produces NADPH which ensures

that glutathione is maintained in a reduced state. Glutathione has –SH (sulfydryl) radicals and these radicals need to be maintained in the reduced state. If the hydrogen from the –SH radicals are lost then S–S (disulfide) bonds take place. This will result in denaturation and precipitation of the protein. NADPH ensures that hydrogen is available to maintain –SH radicals. When the proteins are precipitated they are known as Heinz bodies.

Pyruvate kinase is the commonest enzyme missing in the glycolytic pathway. The condition is transmitted as autosomal recessive. Like any hemolytic anemia, these patients may have anemia, jaundice and gall stones.

68. A

Normally, two isotypes, G6PD-A and G6PD-B, can be differentiated based on electrophoretic mobility. The B isoform is the most common type found in all populations. Approximately 10% of US black men have the G6PD-A minus isoform. The A minus isoform has the same electrophoretic mobility as the A isoform. The A minus form is unstable. This results in loss of enzyme activity. Older RBCs tend to have only 5–15% of original enzyme activity. The other common mutation involving G6PD is the G6PD-Mediterranean. G6PD-A minus variant typically have mild to moderate enzyme deficiency and may produce occasional hemolytic anemia. In contrast, G6PD-Mediterranean form has severe enzyme deficiency and may produce acute hemolytic anemia due to ingestion of drugs or fava beans (referred to as favism). G6PD deficient individuals exhibit bite cells and/or blister cells on the peripheral smear. Heinz bodies are found. However, visualization requires staining by supra vital dyes. G6PD deficiency is typically inherited as X-linked recessive and is the most common enzyme deficiency involving the pentose phosphate pathway.

69. A

PNH is not inherited. It is an acquired disorder due to spontaneous mutation of the phosphatidyl inositol gylcan anchor biosynthesis, class A (PIG-A) gene. The PIG-A gene encodes for cell membrane anchor proteins, referred to as GPI (glcophosphatidyl inositol anchor protein). Some of these anchor proteins regulate complement.

The mutation occurs in pluripotent stem cells. Thus, PNH affects all hematopoietic cells. There occurs increased susceptibility to complement mediated lysis. However, nucleated hematopoietic cells can endocytose membrane attack complexes, thus protecting them from complement mediated lysis. As mature red cells are not nucleated, they are susceptible to lysis.

Examples of missing proteins in PNH are CD55 aka decay accelerating factor (DAF), and CD59 aka membrane inhibitor of reactive lysis (MIRL). CD55 inhibits association of C4b and C2 and also causes dissociation of C4bC2a (aka C3 convertase). CD59 prevents formation of membrane attack complex and thus cell lysis.

Sucrose lysis is a screen test for PNH. Confirmatory tests include Ham's acidified serum test and flow cytometry documenting absence of CD55 and CD59. Ham's acidified serum test can also be positive in congenital dyserythropoietic anemia, type II.

70. C

A true positive Ham's acidified serum test is one in which the patient's red cells will undergo greater than 1% lysis when mixed with patient's own serum and acid is added. Heating to 56 degrees Celsius will destroy complement. Therefore, any tube heated to 56 degrees should not exhibit hemolysis.

71. D

There are three main types of autoimmune hemolytic anemia, WAHA, CHAD and PCH.

In WAHA, the antibodies are typically IgG in nature and often directed against Rh antigens. Hemolysis is extravascular and DAT is positive with IgG or IgG and C3. In CHAD, the antibodies are typically IgM in nature and often directed against the I antigen. Hemolysis if seen is intravascular. DAT is positive for C3. PCH is rare and is sometimes seen in children following a viral infection. Antibodies are IgG in nature and directed against the P antigen. The antibody binds to red cells at low temperature and at higher temperature there occurs complement mediated lysis. The antibody is also known as biphasic antibody or Donath-Landsteiner antibody.

Common causes of WAHA and CHAD include idiopathic, infections (seen more often in CHAD),

drug induced (seen more often in WAHA) and lymphoproliferative states. In WAHA, spherocytes are typically seen on the peripheral smear. In CHAD, red cell agglutination may be seen on the peripheral smear.

72. C

In individuals with HbSS disease, under low oxygen tension, 6 to 8 HbS molecules polymerize to form a tubular structure called tactoid. This distorts the red cells. The red cells when distorted assume the shape of boat cells or sickle cells. Sickle cells can cause occlusion of small vessels, which may result in infarction. Repeated sickling and unsickling results in hemolysis. HbCC disease is characterized by presence of "folded" cells as well as HbC crystals. In HbSC disease abundant target cells are a common feature. Sickle cells, "folded" cells and red cells with HbC crystals may not be seen. If they are present their numbers are significantly less when compared to HbSS disease or HbCC disease.

Target cells are seen in obstructive liver disease, hemoglobinopathies and thalassemia syndromes. They are also seen in deficiency states of lecithin cholesterol acyltransferase (LCAT) deficiency. Occasional target cells may be seen in individuals with iron deficiency. Target cells are formed when there is excess of cell membrane in relation to volume of cytoplasm. In thalassemia and hemoglobiniopathies this is due to reduction in volume of cytoplasm. In obstructive liver disease and LCAT deficiency, target cells are formed due to excess cell membrane lipid.

Macro ovalocytes are a feature of B12 and folate deficiency. Macrocytic anemia due to hypothyroidism, alcohol or liver disease results in red cells with high MCV but macro ovalocytes are not seen.

73. D

Elliptocytes when present in significant numbers (e.g. >20%) may be seen in hereditary elliptocytosis. Other causes include thalassemias and HbAS (sickle cell trait) and HbAC (HbC trait). Occasional elliptocytes may be seen for individuals with iron deficiency, chronic liver disease and megaloblastic anemia.

Stomatocytes are red cells with slit like central pallor. Other than hereditary stomatocytosis, small number of stomatocytes may be seen in individuals with chronic liver disease and Rh null disease.

Echinocytes (also known as "burr cells") are red cells with 10–30 short blunt projections/spicules. They are seen as storage artifact as well as in individuals with liver disease, kidney disease and pyruvate kinase deficiency.

Drepanocytes is another name for sickle cells. Another name for target cells is codocytes.

74. B

The word acanthocyte is derived from the Greek word acantha, meaning thorn. Acanthocytes have 2–20 unequal, irregular thorn like projections. If the majority of red cells are acanthocytes then abetalipoproteinemia is a likely diagnosis. Occasional acanthocytes may be seen in individuals with postsplenectomy, pyruvate kinase deficiency, microangiopathic hemolytic anemia, autoimmune hemolytic anemia and McLeod phenotype. Here the Kx antigen, which is the precursor for the Kell blood group system, is missing. This condition is inherited as an X-linked disorder.

75. A

Howell-Jolly bodies are DNA material and are seen typically as a large RBC inclusion, located peripherally. These bodies may be seen in multiple conditions including, hemolytic states, myelophthisic anemia, megaloblastic anemia and postsplenectomy.

Pappenheimer bodies contain iron and are found within mitochondria. They are seen as multiple bodies, smaller than Howell-Jolly bodies. They may form small, cannon ball-like clusters.

Basophilic stippling is seen due to presence of RNA material. Basophilic stippling if fine may be physiological. Coarse basophilic stippling is typically pathological.

Of all RBC inclusions (e.g. Howell-Jolly bodies, Pappenheimer bodies, Cabot rings, basophilic stippling, Heinz bodies, HbC crystals, Malarial parasites and nucleated RBCs) it is only the HbC crystals which are seen in vitro.

76. B

Pyrimidine 5 nucleotidase is an enzyme responsible for the degradation of RNA. Deficiency will result in basophilic stippling. Lead poisoning results in inhibition of this enzyme, which in turn leads to basophilic stippling.

77. D

Characteristic features of red cells infested with Plasmodium falciparum are:

1. Red cells are not enlarged
2. Delicate ring forms of Plasmodium falciparum with more than one ring per red cell
3. Ring forms with two chromatin dots
4. Presence of marginal (aka appliqué) forms; this is where the parasite appears to be present on the surface of red cells
5. Banana- or crescent-shaped gametocytes
6. Developing forms not seen
7. Maurer's dots may be seen

78. D

In CHAD the antibody is typically IgM in nature. There is an association with Mycoplasma pneumoniae infection. Red cell agglutination is an in vitro phenomenon. When red cell agglutination takes place the analyzer counts a clump of red cell as one red cell. Thus the red cell count will be low. The MCV value will be falsely high. However, when the red cells are lysed to obtain hemoglobin values, an accurate value will be obtained.

79. D

Microangiopathic hemolysis is characterized by presence of fragmented red cells (schistocytes) and thrombocytopenia in the peripheral blood. In DIC coagulation, parameters such as PT and PTT are abnormal and prolonged. In contrast in TTP and HUS, coagulation parameters such as PT and PTT are essentially normal.

80. A

Increase in MCHC is a characteristic finding in hereditary spherocytosis. The MCV and MCH are usually normal. The reticulocyte count, bilirubin and LDH are all elevated. Review of the peripheral smear demonstrates spherocytes (red cells with no central pallor).

81. D

Hereditary spherocytosis is usually transmitted as autosomal dominant but in some families it may be transmitted as autosomal recessive. Also 20% of cases are due to spontaneous mutation.

G6PD deficiency is transmitted as X-linked recessive and like other X-linked recessive conditions may be seen in females with homozygosity, asymmetric lyonization and in patients who have Turner's syndrome. Pyruvate kinase deficiency is transmitted as autosomal recessive. Rarely, in AML and MDS it may be acquired.

PK deficiency typically causes chronic hemolysis in contrast to G6PD deficiency where hemolysis tends to be episodic.

82. B

The sensitivity and specificity for the EMA binding test is the highest, followed closely by the AGLT. Combining the two tests allows detection of virtually all cases of hereditary spherocytosis.

Osmotic Fragility Testing

Spherocytes are prone to osmotic lysis in hypotonic solutions. This is the basis for the osmotic fragility test, which detects hemolysis by measuring the fraction of total hemoglobin released from red cells at progressively more dilute salt concentrations. Incubation of blood for 24 hours in the absence of metabolic substrate increases the sensitivity of the test.

Acidified Glycerol Lysis Test

Here, red blood cells are incubated in a phosphate buffered hypotonic solution with added glycerol, which slows the entrance of water into the cells. Spherocytes from patients with hereditary spherocytosis lyse more quickly than normal red blood cells

Eosin-5-maleimide Binding Test

This is a a flow cytometric test. It is based on the interaction between the dye eosin-5-maleimide and band 3 protein. Only small volumes of red cells are required (5 to 10 microL), the test can be performed on capillary blood.

Eosin-5-maleimide binds to several red cell proteins, including band 3, Rh polypeptides and CD 47. Reduction in the amount of one or more of these membrane proteins in several forms of HS (eg, spectrin deficiency, band 3 deficiency) accounts for the high predictive value of this screening. Mild cases of HS may not always be detected, and false positive results may be obtained in congenital dyserythropoietic anemia type II and occasionally in autoimmune hemolytic anemia.

83. D

Cryoglobulins are immunoglobulins that precipitate at low temperatures. There are three types of cryoglobulinema, types I, II and III. In type I cyroglobulinemia the immunoglobulins are monoclonal and this condition is seen in association with multiple myeloma or Waldenstroms' macroglobulinemia. In type II cryoglobulinemia there is a mixture of monoclonal IgM and polyclonal IgG immunoglobulins. This type is the most common type seen. In type III there is only polyclonal immunoglobulins. An individual may also have mixed type (types II and type III). HCV infection is the most common cause of mixed cryoglobulinemia. Mixed cryoglobulinemia is most common in women in their 4th and 5th decades. Underlying causes include chronic liver disease, chronic infections, autoimmune diseases and lymphroliferative disorders.

Clinically, patients with cryoglobulinemia develop features such as purpura (due to vasculitic lesions of skin), arthralgia, anemia, glomerulonephritis, lymphadenopathy and hepatosplenomegaly.

84. C

Spurious erythrocytosis seen in individuals with dehydration is referred to as Gaisbock syndrome.

85. D

During the embryonic stage, hemoglobin Gower and hemoglobin Portland predominates. During the fetal life, the major hemoglobin is hemoglobin F. During the third trimester, hemoglobin A and A2 start to appear. Newborns continue to have significant levels of hemoglobin F till 6 months of age. After one year of age hemoglobin F is typically less than 1%, hemoglobin A is less than 3.5% and the remainder is hemoglobin A.

Hemoglobin A contains two α chains and two β chains. The normal α chain has 141 amino acids and the normal β chain has 146 amino acids. Hemoglobin A2 contains two α chains and two δ chains. Hemoglobin F contains two α chains and two γ chains. The gene for the α chains resides in chromosome 16. The genes for the β, γ and δ chains reside in chromosome 11.

86. D

Hemoglobin adducts are post-translational modifications of hemoglobin molecules. When glucose is added to hemoglobin A, it is known as HbA1c. Similarly individuals with HbS and HbC will have HbS1c and HbC1c, respectively. When the hemoglobin molecule is aged, glutathione becomes bound to cysteine at the 93 rd position of the β chain. When this occurs to HbA, this is known as HbA1d or HbAIII. Similarly, patients can have HbS1d and HbC1d, if they have HbS and HbC respectively.

Hemoglobin Constant Spring is not a hemoglobin adduct. It is an abnormal hemoglobin that may be seen in individuals with α thalassemia.

87. B

The first step in the hemoglobin biosynthetic pathway is formation of δ aminolevulinic acid from glycine and succinyl CoA, which takes place in the mitochondria. δ aminolevulinic acid is transported to the cytoplasm where it is converted to porphobilinogen. Porphobilinogen is converted to coproporphyrinogen III, which in turn is converted to protoporphyrinogen III in the mitochondria. This is converted to protoporphyrin IX and then to heme by the enzyme ferrochelatase. Here iron is added, not withdrawn. The heme is transported back to the cytoplasm to combine with globin chains to form hemoglobin.

88. B

There are over 1,000 hemoglobinopathies described. Thankfully, most are asymptomatic. About 5% of the population in the world are carriers of hemoglobinopathies. Thalassemias are characterized by reduced amount of globin chain synthesis. The globin chains are structurally normal. Hemoglobinopathies are characterized by abnormal globins.
Individuals with HbC are most likely of western African ancestry.

89. D

HbSS, HbSC, HbSD and HbSO are all sickling disorders. HbSE is not a sickling disorder.

90. C

Carriers of α thalassemia have three functional α genes. The fourth α gene is defective or deleted. In some carriers, there are three functional α genes and there is Hb Constant Spring (HbCS) being produced from the fourth mutated α gene. HbCS is the result of a nondeletion mutation of the α gene. It is underproduced and is unstable.

HbCS has an abnormally long α chain and has 172 aminoacids. It is named after the Constant Spring district in Jamaica where it was first isolated.

Individuals with α thalassemia trait have two functional α genes. These individuals may have mild microcytic hypochromic anemia.

HbH is characterized by presence of one functional α gene. These individuals have significant anemia.

When there is loss of all α genes, then the baby typically dies in utero and the condition is also known as hydrops fetalis.

91. A

α thalassemia occurs when there is deletion of two α genes. There are two forms of α thalassemia trait. If due to alpha thalassemia 1 (-/-, α, α), which is due to cis deletion of both α genes on the same chromosome, is seen more often in the Southeast Asian population. If due to α thalassemia 2 (-/ α, -/α), which is due to trans deletion of the α genes on two different chromosomes, is seen more often in the African and African American population. Patients are largely asymptomatic. There may be mild microcytic hypochromic anemia. Thus it may mimic iron deficiency anemia.

92. D

In α thalassemia, there is significant underproduction of α chains. In such states, four γ chains, which are present in the newborn will combine to form a novel hemoglobin, Hb Bart's. Later on in life, when β chains are produced instead of γ chains, four α chains will form the HbH. Thus, adults with α thalassemia disease will have HbH. HbH has high affinity for oxygen and thus there will be tissue hypoxemia. HbH is sensitive to oxidative stress and is more susceptible to hemolysis.
HbH may be precipitated and will result in formation of Heinz bodies. Patients have chronic hemolytic anemia. Red cells are microcytic and hypochromic with presence of target cells. There is widespread erythroid hyperplasia with subsequent bony structural abnormalities.

93. B

Individuals with β thalassemia have elevated HbA2. Normally, HbA2 is less than 3.5%. In β thalassemia trait HbF may or may not be elevated. All individuals with β thalassemia typically have microcytic hypochromic red cells with target cells in the peripheral smear. In β thalassemia trait anemia is mild and patients do not require transfusion. In β thalassemia major, when both β chains are defective, there is no production of HbA. Thus, all the hemoglobins are HbA2 and HbF. Anemia is severe and requires regular blood transfusion. In β thalassemia, intermedia features are in between β thalassemia trait and beta thalassemia major. Patients may require transfusion from time to time. Here, although both β chains are defective, some β globin chain production is possible. Thus, the patient has some HbA.

94. D

α thalassemia trait and iron deficiency anemia are causes of low HbA2 levels. Thus if an individual has iron deficiency with β thalassemia trait, low levels of HbA2 due to iron deficiency may mask the diagnosis of β thalassemia trait. It may be necessary to repeat hemoglobin electrophoresis after the iron deficiency has been corrected. δ thalassemia is due to mutation of the gene for δ chain. If delta chain production is zero, then HbA2 levels are undetectable. If δ chain production is lower than normal, then HbA2 levels are low. Again, if δ and β thalassemia co-exist, detection of β thalassemia trait may be difficult due to low levels of HbA2.

95. C

β thalassemia trait individuals should have elevated HbA2 levels. β thalassemia major individuals typically have elevated HbF and elevated HbA2 levels. Although at times an individual with β thalassemia major may not demonstrate elevated HbA2 levels. In either situation, β thalassemia major patients do not have HbA (unless transfused) and have very high levels of HbF. Individuals with δ thalassemia have low levels of HbA2. In this case, levels of HbA2 are normal, not low.

In δ β thalassemia there is decreased production of delta and beta globin chains. HbA2 levels are normal. HbF is increased and typically between 5% and 15%. Delta beta thalassemia is found more often in individuals who are of Greek or Italian ancestry. Heterozygous individuals are largely asymptomatic.

96. D

A represents the defect seen in HbE.
B represents the defect seen in HbO
C represents the defect seen in HbC.

All are β chain defects. In all glutamic acid is replaced by lysine, except in HbS where glutamic acid is replaced by valine.

97. D

Patients with HbSS disease may have increased HbF. The distribution of HbF among the haplotypes of HbSS are HbF 5–7% in Bantu, Benin, or Cameroon; Hb F 7–10% in Senegal; and HbF 10–25% in Arab-Indian.

Hydroxyurea also causes an increase in HbF. This is usually accompanied by macrocytosis. HbF can also be increased in HbS/HPFH (hereditary persistence of fetal hemoglobin).

98. A

HbSS disease and HbS/β zero thalassemia can result in severe sickling disorders. HbSC gives rise to a milder sickling disorder than the above two conditions. Overall, it is generally considered to be a moderate sickling disorder. HbS/HPFH typically produces a mild sickling disorder. Individuals with sickle cell trait do not have sickling disorders.

99. C

HbD (Punjab, Los Angeles and Iran) and Hb E when present are produced in abundant quantities (i.e. approximately 30% in heterozygous states). Hb Lepore, Hb Constant Spring (HbCS) and HbA2' are three abnormal hemoglobins which are typically produced in low quantities.

Hb Lepore is an unusual hemoglobin, which is formed from two α chains and two δ β chains. This occurs due to fusion of the δ and β genes. The δ β chain will consist of the first 87 amino acids of the δ chain and 32 aminoacids of the β chain. Individuals who are heterozygous for Hb Lepore will have 5–15% of Hb Lepore with mild increase in HbF (2–3%). The remainder will be HbA.

100. C

Physiological causes of elevated levels of HbF are young age (newborns and children up to one year of age) and pregnancy. In pregnancy HbF levels can increase up to 5%. Important pathological causes of elevated HbF include:

1. β thalassemia (Here HbA2 is high and the red cells are microcytic and hypochromic)

2. δ β thalassemia trait (Here HbF is typically between 5 and 15%; HbA2 is not increased and the patient has microcytic hypochromic red cells)

3. In association with HbSS disease with or without hydroxyurea therapy

4. HbS/β thalassemia

5. Hb Lepore

6. Hematologic conditions such as aplastic anemia, acute erythroid leukemia, juvenile myelomonocytic leukemia

101. D

Hbs J, I N, Bart's and HbH are all examples of fast hemoglobin on alkaline agarose gel electrophoresis. On the alkaline they all travel beyond the A lane. However, Hbs J, I and N are typically clinically insignificant. Hbs Bart's and HbH are typically seen in individuals with α thalassemia.

102. D

HbS, is a β chain defect, and is most often seen in African American individuals. HbG is the most common α chain defect. It is also most often seen in African American individuals. An individual with HbS/HbG disease will have the following hemoglobins:

1. HbA (normal α chains and normal β chains)

2. HbS (normal α chain but defective β chain

3. HbG (abnormal α chain and normal β chain)

4. HbS/HbG (abnormal α and β chains)

5. HbG2, which is the counterpart of HbA2

On alkaline gel there will be three distinct bands and one faint band (if too faint may not be obvious).

The three distinct bands are: one band in the C lane due to HbS/HbG hybrid; one band in the S lane due to HbS and HbG; one band in the A lane due to HbA. HbG2 may be seen as a faint band in the carbonic anhydrase area.

On acid gel there will be two distinct bands: one band in the S lane due to HbS and HbS/HbG hybrid, and one band in the A lane due to HbA and HbG.

103. A

With HPLC, carryover of a specimen to the next is an established problem.

104. C

Transfusion history is always important in interpreting hemoglobin electrophoresis results. Apparent hemoglobinopathy after blood transfusion is a well recognized phenomenon. Patients with HbS trait and HbC trait are both allowed to donate blood. Post-transfusion electrophoresis may cause diagnostic confusion. Typically the abnormal hemoglobin from the donor is present at low levels (0.8–14%, median 5.6%).

105. A

In methemoglobinemia there is higher than normal level of methemoglobin (Hi). Normally, methemoglobin levels are less than 1%. In methemoglobin, the iron is in the ferric form (Fe^{3+}). Methemoglobinemia results in increased oxygen binding to hemoglobin. Less oxygen is released to the tissues. This results in tissue hypoxia and cyanosis. With methemoglobinemia the color of the blood is blue or chocolate brown. Methemoglobin levels are measured by the co-oximetry test. There are two forms of methemoglobinemia, congenital and acquired. Congenital methemoglobinemia may be due to deficiency of the enzyme NADH-cytochrome-b5 reductase (also known as NADH methemoglobin reductase). This is transmitted as autosomal recessive. In this condition methemoglobin cannot be reduced back to Hb. Another cause of congenital methemoglobinemia is HbM. Here the enzyme system is intact. Acquired causes of methemoglobinemia is typically due to drugs. Examples include antibiotics (e.g. trimethoprim, sulfonamides, dapsone), and local anesthetics. Ingestion of compounds containing nitrates can also cause methemoglobinemia.

106. B

Individuals with sickle cell disease undergo autosplenectomy during adolescent years. Thus when they are adults the peripheral smear may exhibit target cells, acanthocytes and

Howell-Jolly bodies. These findings are common to individuals who have undergone splenectomy or autosplenectomy. Two important causes of autosplenectomy are sickle cell disease and celiac disease.

107. B

Methemoglobin (Hi) is hemoglobin where the iron is in the ferric state (Fe+++). Hi cannot bind with oxygen. Normally levels of Hi are low (up to 1.5%). Low levels are maintained by the enzyme methemoglobin reductase. Causes of elevated Hi include hereditary and acquired causes. Examples of hereditary causes of methemoglobinemia are deficiency of the enzyme methemoglobin reductase and abnormal hemoglobins (HbM). Methemoglobin reductase cannot act upon these abnormal HbMs. Examples of such hemoglobins include Hb M-Boston and HbM-Saskatoon. With elevated levels of Hi, cyanosis is an expected finding.

108. D

Sickle cell disease, sickle cell trait and HbSC disease all are associated with increased risk of medullary carcinoma of the kidneys.

109. D

High oxygen affinity hemoglobin such as Hb Chesapeake will result in a leftward shift of the oxygen dissociation curve. Low oxygen affinity hemoglobin such as Hb Beth Israel will result in a rightward shift of the oxygen dissociation curve. Most of these altered oxygen affinity hemoglobins cannot be detected by gel electrophoresis or HPLC. Analysis of the oxygen dissociation curve is useful.

Unstable hemoglobins will result in precipitation of the abnormal hemoglobin if lysed red cells are incubated with 17% isopropanol. Thus these group of hemoglobins will result in Heinz bodies and bite cells, similar to G6PD deficiency. Oxidative stress will result in hemolytic episodes.

Non-Neoplastic WBC and Platelet Disorders

WBC and Platelet Disorders: Questions 1–15

1. Pelger-Huet anomaly is characterized by:
   A. Increased incidence of bacterial infections
   B. Transmission as autosomal dominant
   C. Dohle like bodies in the neutrophil cytoplasm
   D. 10% of neutrophils with bilobed nucleus

2. Alder-Reilly anomaly is characterized by:
   A. Increased incidence of bacterial infections
   B. Transmission as autosomal recessive
   C. Dohle like bodies in the neutrophil cytoplasm
   D. Large azurophilic granules only in neutrophils

3. May-Hegglin anomaly is characterized by:
   A. Small platelets
   B. Transmission as autosomal recessive
   C. Dohle like bodies in the neutrophil cytoplasm
   D. Toxic granulation of the neutrophil cytoplasm

4. All of the following are true regarding Chediak-Higashi syndrome except:
   A. Transmission as autosomal dominant
   B. Hypopigmentation of skin
   C. Increased incidence of lymphoproliferative disorder
   D. Lysosomal inclusion bodies in WBCs

5. All of the following are causes of neutrophilic leukocytosis except:
   A. Cushing's syndrome
   B. Addison's disease
   C. Bacterial infection
   D. Rheumatoid arthritis

6. A low leukocyte alkaline phosphatase score is expected in:
   A. Polycythemia vera
   B. Acute myeloid leukemia

   C. Essential thrombocythemia
   D. Chronic myeloid leukemia

7. All of the following regarding neutropenia are true except:
   A. Cyclical neutropenia is typically characterized by neutropenia occurring every three weeks
   B. Kostmann's syndrome is transmitted as autosomal dominant
   C. Neutropenia is a feature of Felty's syndrome
   D. If neutropenia is due to Shwachmann-Diamond syndrome, there is associated exocrine pancreatic deficiency

8. Regarding lymphocytosis and reactive lymphocytes or Downey cells:
   A. Type I Downey cells which are reactive lymphocytes with abundant pale blue cytoplasm are the most common type
   B. In infectious mononucleosis, only one type of reactive lymphocytes is seen
   C. Rarely seen with bacterial infections; however, infection due to Bordetella pertussis is an exception
   D. Easily distinguished from lymphoid leukemias in all cases

9. The disease condition which results due to mutation of the WASP gene is:
   A. Kasabach-Meritt syndrome
   B. Wiskott-Aldrich syndrome
   C. May-Hegglin anomaly
   D. Benard Soulier syndrome

10. All of the following are causes of small platelets except:
   A. Wiskott-Aldrich syndrome
   B. X-linked thrombocytopenia

C. Autosomal dominant, inherited microthrombocytes

D. Bernard Soulier syndrome

11. Which of the following statements is incorrect?

A. Bernard Soulier syndrome is transmitted as autosomal recessive

B. Glanzmann's thrombasthenia is characterized by giant platelets

C. Bernard Soulier syndrome patients show impaired aggregation to high dose of ristocetin

D. Some cases of Bernard Soulier syndrome are due to defects of the GpIb β gene, located on chromosome 22

12. All of the following are disorders due to defective myosin heavy chain 9 gene located at 22q11, except:

A. May-Hegglin anomaly

B. Sebastian syndrome

C. Epstein syndrome

D. Gray platelet syndrome

13. All of the following are examples of secondary thrombocytosis except:

A. Familial thrombocytosis

B. Iron deficiency

C. Rheumatoid arthritis

D. Post-splenectomy

14. All of the following are established causes of thrombocytopathia (platelet dysfunction) except:

A. Uremia

B. Clopidogrel

C. Coumadin

D. Essential thrombocythemia

15. Regarding reactive lymphocytes (aka Downey cells):

A. A cell, larger than the usual lymphocyte, with abundant cytoplasm that surrounds (or "hugs") the red cells (known as Downey Type II cells) are the most common type of reactive lymphocytes

B. Presence of reactive lymphocytes should trigger search for an underlying lymphoproliferative disorder

C. Usually seen with bacterial infections in adults

D. Have a unique immunophenotype

Answers to Chapter 2

1. B
2. B
3. C
4. A

5. B
6. D
7. B
8. C

9. B
10. D
11. B
12. D

13. A
14. C
15. A

Answers to Chapter 2 (with Explanations)

1. B

   Pelger-Huet anomaly is a benign condition in which the vast majority of neutrophils (>75%) have a bilobed nucleus. It is transmitted as autosomal dominant. An inherited defect of terminal neutrophil differentiation occurs. This is due to mutations in the laminin B receptor (LBR) gene. Occasional presence of neutrophils similar to Pelger-Huet cells may be seen in individuals with myelodysplastic syndrome. These cells are referred to as pseudo Pelger-Huet cells.

2. B

   Alder-Reilly is another benign condition where large azurophilic granules are seen in the cytoplasm of granulocytes as well as lymphocytes and monocytes. The granules correspond to partially degraded protein-carbohydrate complexes. The condition is transmitted as autosomal recessive. Similar morphology may be seen in mucopolysaccharidoses.

3. C

   May-Hegglin anomaly is characterized by thrombocytopenia, giant platelets and the presence of Dohle like bodies in neutrophil cytoplasm. Actual Dohle bodies are seen in the cytoplasm of reactive neutrophils. Reactive neutrophils will also exhibit other features of reactive changes. These include toxic granulation and cytoplasmic vacuoles. May-Hegglin anomaly does not exhibit these features. Transmission is autosomal dominant. Small platelets are seen in the Wiskott-Aldrich syndrome.

4. A

   Chediak-Higashi syndrome is a rare multisystemic disease, transmitted as autosomal recessive. The WBCs are filled with massive lysosomal inclusion bodies. Leukocyte function is impaired with immunodeficiency. There is increased incidence of lymphoreticular malignancies, especially in childhood. This is a potentially fatal condition if left untreated.

5. B

   There are multiple causes of neutrophilia. These include

   1. Infection, especially bacterial infection
   2. Inflammatory states (e.g. Rheumatoid arthritis)
   3. High levels of glucocorticoids (e.g. iatrogenic, Cushing's syndrome)
   4. Acute blood loss
   5. Hemolysis
   6. Postsplenectomy states
   7. Rare causes: hereditary neutrophilia, idiopathic neutrophilia, leukocyte adhesion deficiency

6. D.

   Significant neutrophilic leukocytosis with left shift is termed as leukemoid reaction. The condition may resemble chronic myeloid leukemia (CML). There will be key differences between leukemoid reaction and CML. For example, leukemoid reaction should exhibit reactive/toxic changes. There should be basophilia and eosinophilia in CML. In the recent past leukocyte alkaline phosphatase score was done to help differentiate the two conditions. In this test, neutrophils are stained for alkaline phosphatase. Each neutrophil is given a score from 0 to 4 based on the intensity of staining. One hundred cells are counted. In CML the score is expected to be very low. In other myeloproliferative conditions as well as leukemoid reactions scores are not low. paroxysmal nocturnal hemoglobinuria (PNH) is another condition where LAP score is low.

7. B

   Neutropenia is a condition where the neutrophil count is more than two standard deviations below the normal count. Mild neutropenia may be asymptomatic. However, neutrophil counts below

500/mm³ can result in significant infections which can be life threatening.

Causes of neutropenia include:

1. Drugs
2. Infection
3. Autoimmune
4. Splenomegaly
5. Felty's syndrome
6. paroxysmal nocturnal hemoglobinuria (PNH)
7. Cyclical neutropenia: here neutropenia occurs approximately every three weeks. There is also a familial form of this condition, transmitted as autosomal dominant.
8. Kostmann's syndrome: this is transmitted as autosomal recessive. Here occurs a mutation in the gene coding for the granulocyte colony stimulating factor.
9. Shwachmann-Diamond syndrome: here occurs neutropenia, thrombocytopenia, short stature, mental retardation and exocrine pancreatic insufficiency. This disorder is known to progress to myelodysplastic syndrome and acute myeloid leukemia.

8. C

Lymphocytosis typically accompanies viral infections; however, infection due to Bordetella pertussis is an exception. Reactive lymphocytes aka Downey cells may accompany lymphocytosis. There are three types of Downey cells:

I: these are small cells with indented/irregular nuclei, condensed nuclear chromatin, and minimal cytoplasm.

II: these are the most common type of Downey cells. These cells have abundant pale blue cytoplasm which surrounds and appears to "hug" adjacent red blood cells.

III: these cells have basophilic cytoplasm and prominent nucleoli.

Downey cells, especially types I and III, may resemble cells seen in the blood with lymphoid leukemias.

In infectious mononucleosis, review of the peripheral blood may show characteristic features which are:

A. Presence of 50% or more of mononuclear cells among the white cells

B. 10% or more of the lymphocytes are reactive

C. The same patient has different types of Downey cells at the same time. This is referred to as lymphocytic morphologic heterogeneity.

9. B

The WASP gene is located at Xp11. Mutation results in Wiskott Aldrich syndrome. Inheritance is X-linked recessive. Patients have thrombocytopenia, dysfunctional platelets, small platelets, eczema and immunodeficiency.

Kasabach-Meritt syndrome is thrombocytopenia in association with a hemangioma.

10. D

Wiskott Aldrich syndrome has been discussed previously. X-linked thrombocytopenia is a congenital disorder where isolated thrombocytopenia with small platelets occurs. No other clinical features are evident. Inherited microthrombocytes is another condition where there is thrombocytopenia but with normal platelet function. It is transmitted as autosomal dominant.

Bernard Soulier syndrome is characterized by thrombocytopenia with large and giant platelets.

11. B

Bernard Souiler syndrome is characterized by thrombocytopenia and macrothrombocytes. Here the GpIb-V-IX complex is abnormal. Inheritance is autosomal recessive. Platelet aggregation demonstrates impaired aggregation to high-dose ristocetin. Some cases of Bernard Soulier syndrome are due to defects of the β gene, located on chromosome 22. This gene may be affected in velocardiofacial syndrome or Di George syndrome associated with the deletion of 22q11.2

Glanzmann's thrombasthenia is due to the abnormality of GpIIb/IIIa complex. Inheritance is also autosomal recessive. There is normal aggregation with ristocetin. However, there is failure of aggregation to other agonists such as arachidonic acid, ADP, collagen and epinephrine. Glanzmann's thrombasthenia is not characterized by giant platelets.

12. D

May-Hegglin anomaly, Sebastian syndrome, Epstein syndrome and Fechtner syndrome are all conditions associated with defective myosin heavy chain nine gene located at 22q11. They are all transmitted as autosomal dominant. In all, neutrophils have Dohle like bodies.

Gray platelet syndrome is transmitted as autosomal recessive. Platelets are devoid of alpha granules. These granules are stained by Wright giemsa stain. Absence of the granules makes the platelets appear gray. Patients have a tendency to bleed. In contrast, absence of delta granules cannot be picked up by routine peripheral smear. Electron microscopy is required to document their absence.

13. A

Familial thrombocytosis is due to a mutation in the thrombopoietin receptor gene. It is transmitted as autosomal dominant. Causes of secondary thrombocytosis include infections, inflammatory states, iron deficiency, neoplasms and postsplenectomy states.

14. C

Thrombocytopathia may be categorized into congenital and acquired causes.

Congenital thrombocytopathia:

1. Disorders of platelet adhesion: Von Willebrand's disease, Bernard Soulier syndrome

2. Disorders of platelet activation: Chediak Higashi syndrome, storage pool disorders, Hermansky Pudlak syndrome

3. Disorders of platelet aggregation: Glanzmann's thrombasthenia

Acquired thrombocytopathia:

1. Uremia
2. Antiplatelet drugs, e.g., aspirin, clopidogrel
3. Acquired Von Willebrand's disease
4. Hypofibrinogenemia
5. Myeloproliferative disorders
6. Autoimmune: antiplatelet antibodies

15. A

Reactive lymphocytes are of three types: Downey I, II and III.

Downey type II cells are the most common. They are cells larger than a mature lymphocyte and with abundant cytoplasm. The reactive lymphocytes appear to hug the red cells. Downey type I cell is a cell with nuclear membrane irregularity. Downey type III cells are large lymphocytes with blue cytoplasm and nucleoli. Downey type I and III cells may resemble atypical lymphocytes. Atypical lymphocytes are generally considered to be lymphocytes which are suspicious for underlying lymphoproliferative disorders.

Benign Lymph Node

Benign Lymph Node: Questions 1–16

1. Regarding a normal secondary follicle in a lymph node:
   A. The outer mantle zone stains for CD3 and CD5
   B. Outer to the mantle zone is the marginal zone which is a T-cell area
   C. The light zone in the germinal centre consists of centrocytes, where the mitotic rate is high
   D. The dark zone consists of centroblasts with a high mitotic rate

2. Features that support follicular hyperplasia, rather than follicular lymphoma, are:
   A. Uniform follicles which are back to back
   B. Indistinct mantle zone
   C. Bcl-2 negative within the germinal center
   D. Loss of polarity in the germinal center

3. Which of the following features are strongly suggestive of viral lymphadenopathy?
   A. Marked follicular hyperplasia
   B. Paracortical hyperplasia with a mottled appearance
   C. Diffuse effacement of the lymph node architecture with sheets of large cells
   D. Presence of Reed Sternberg cells

4. All of the following are true about HIV lymphadenopathy except:
   A. Lymph node findings correlate with CD4 status in the peripheral blood
   B. Three different patterns may be seen (patterns A, B and C)
   C. Warthin Finkeldey giant cells may be seen
   D. Follicular hyperplasia is typically seen

5. Regarding lymph node histology of cat scratch disease:
   A. Warthin Starry stain will highlight the bacteria Bartonella henselae
   B. Paracortical hyperplasia is the most common finding
   C. Increased eosinophils are typically seen
   D. Granulomas are not an expected finding

6. Regarding Toxoplasma gondii infection and lymphadenopathy, all of the following are true except:
   A. Toxoplasma gondii is an extracellular protozoan
   B. Humans may be infected from contact with cat feces
   C. Primary infection with Toxoplasma gondii during pregnancy may result in congenital toxoplasmosis
   D. Toxoplasma lymphadenopathy is characterized by follicular hyperplasia, clusters of epithelioid histicocytes and clusters of monocytoid B-cells

7. Microscopic examination of an enlarged lymph node demonstrates dilatation of sinuses with large lipid vacuoles. Multinucleated giant cells are noted within the sinuses. Macrophages are seen with vacuolated cytoplasm. Bacteria are identified within these macrophages which are PAS positive (and diastase resistant). The most likely diagnosis is lymphadenopathy due to:
   A. Actinomyces
   B. Staphylococcus
   C. Tropheryma whipplei
   D. Treponema pallidum

8. An example of granulomatous lymphadenopathy due to noninfectious cause includes:
   A. Tularemia
   B. Cat scratch disease
   C. Tuberculosis
   D. Rheumatoid arthritis

9. A 32-year-old Asian female develops painless cervical lymphadenopathy. An excisional biopsy is performed and histology demonstrates necrotic areas in the paracortex with the presence of karyorrhectic debris. The necrotic areas contain eosinophilic fibrinoid deposits. The necrotic areas are surrounded by numerous histiocytes. Neutrophils are absent. These findings are most consistent with:
   A. Progressive transformation of germinal centers
   B. Cat scratch disease
   C. Kikuchi-Fujimoto disease
   D. Tuberculosis

10. A 20-year-old Asian male has eosinophilia and high levels of IgE with cervical lymphadenopathy. Excisional biopsy of the lymph node demonstrates follicular hyperplasia, intense eosinophilia and eosinophilic microabscesses. The most likely diagnosis is:
    A. Kimura disease
    B. Kikuchi-Fujimoto disease
    C. Eosinophilic leukemia
    D. Hypereosinophilic syndrome

11. Regressive changes in the germinal centers may be seen in:
    A. Castleman disease
    B. HIV/AIDS
    C. Postradiation
    D. All of the above

12. Paracortical hyperplasia with macrophages containing brown melanin pigment in lymph nodes draining areas of skin involved with inflammation is a feature of:
    A. Kawasaki disease
    B. Dermatopathic lymphadenitis
    C. Melanoma
    D. Sarcoidosis

13. Which of the following is true for Rosai Dorfman disease?
    A. The disease presents as painful inguinal lymphadenopathy

B. Recovery requires intensive chemotherapy
C. Histology demonstrates marked prominence of eosinophils
D. Histology demonstrates emperipolesis

14. Langerhans Cell Histiocytosis differs from Rosai Dorfman disease in all of the following points except:
    A. The Langerhans cells and the macrophages seen in Rosai Dorfman are CD68 positive
    B. CD1a is positive in Langerhans cell histiocytosis but negative in Rosai Dorfman disease
    C. Eosinophils are typically present in Langerhans cell histiocytosis but not in Rosai Dorfman disease
    D. Langerhans cells have nuclear grooves, a feature not seen within the macrophages of Rosai Dorfman disease

15. A patient with lymphadenopathy undergoes excisional biopsy for further evaluation. Histology demonstrates follicular hyperplasia. The germinal centers are depleted of lymphocytes. Hyaline deposits are present within the germinal centers. The mantle zone is expanded. Sclerotic blood vessels are seen penetrating the follicles. The most likely diagnosis is:
    A. Castleman disease
    B. Mantle cell lymphoma
    C. Sarcoidosis
    D. Regressive changes in germinal centers

16. All of the following are true about Castleman disease except:
    A. Castleman disease is associated with HHV-8 infection
    B. Castleman disease is associated with EBV infection
    C. Castleman disease may predispose to follicular dendritic cell sarcoma
    D. Castleman disease may predispose to malignant lymphoma

Answers to Chapter 3

1.	D	5.	A	9.	C	13.	D
2.	C	6.	A	10.	A	14.	A
3.	B	7.	C	11.	D	15.	A
4.	A	8.	D	12.	B	16.	B

Answers to Chapter 3 (with Explanations)

1. D

   Secondary follicles are derived from primary follicles after antigenic stimulation. The primary follicles consists of naïve B-cells that move into the germinal centers when stimulated. The naïve B-cells transform into centroblasts, which in turn form centrocytes. The centrocytes further differentiate into plasma cells and memory B-cells. Plasma cells move to the medulla. Memory cells reside in the marginal zone.

   Secondary follicles consist of an outer mantle zone and an inner germinal center. The germinal center of a reactive follicle has a light zone and a dark zone. This is referred to as polarity. Within the light zone are centrocytes and follicular dendritic cells. The mitotic rate is low. Tingible body macrophages which are responsible for cleaning up of cells are also low in this area. The dark zone consists of centroblasts with a high mitotic rate and more tangible body macrophages.

   The germinal center of a reactive follicle stains for CD10 and Bcl-6. It is negative for Bcl-2.

2. C

   Table 3.1 contrasts common findings in follicular lymphoma versus reactive follicular hyperplasia.

Follicular lymphoma	Follicular hyperplasia
Back-to-back follicles. The follicles are of uniform size	Follicle are of various size
Indistinct mantle zone	Distinct mantle zone
Loss of polarity	Polarity maintained
Germinal center lacks tingible body macrophages	Germinal center has tingible body macrophages (unless grade III)
Lymphocytes extend beyond capsule	Lymphocytes do not extend beyond capsule
Low Ki-67 unless grade III	High K1-67 in the germinal centers
Bcl-2 positive in the germinal centers	Bcl-2 negative in the germinal centers

3. B

   Viral lymphadenopathy typically results in paracortical hyperplasia. There is also hyperplasia of the interdigitating dendritic cells. These cells have pale cytoplasm. This gives the paracortex a mottled appearance. Follicular hyperplasia, is not a characteristic finding, but may be present in some cases. Reactive lymphocytes that have undergone transformation to larger cells, termed "immunoblasts," may also be seen. These immunoblasts may mimic large cell lymphoma. Reed-Sternberg like cells may also be present.

4. A

   HIV lymphadenopathy typically shows three histopathologic patterns (Patterns A, B, and C). Pattern A is the early pattern where as pattern C is the late pattern. Pattern A shows florid follicular hyperplasia, often with decreased or absent mantle zones, and large germinal centers showing irregular, serpiginous, or "dumb-bell" shaped morphology. There are also folliculolysis and interfollicular hemorrhage. There is also aggregates of monocytoid B-cells. Warthin Finkeldey giant cells may be evident. In pattern C, the follicles are atrophic. There is vascular proliferation. Lollipop appearance of follicles similar to those seen in Castleman disease may be seen. Pattern B has mixed features of pattern A and C.

5. A

   Cat scratch disease typically results in follicular hyperplasia with necrosis and acute inflammation. Areas of necrosis are surrounded by palisading histiocytes. Giant cells may also be seen. Warthin Starry stain will highlight the bacteria, Bartonella henselae.

6. A

   Toxoplasma gondii is an intracellular protozoan and is capable of infecting many species as well as humans. Contact with cat feces infected with Toxoplasma gondii is a common mode of infection for humans. Primary infection during pregnancy may result in congenital toxoplasmosis of the baby, still birth or spontaneous abortion. Toxoplasma lymphadenopathy is characterized by a triad of histologic findings. These are follicular hyperplasia, clusters of epithelioid macrophages in or around germinal centers and clusters of monocytoid B-cells within sinuses.

7. C

The description provided is most consistent with lymphadenopathy due to Tropheryma whipplei.

Lymphadenopathy due to staphylococcus and streptococcus demonstrates features of acute inflammation with necrosis. Abscess formation may also be seen. Subsequently there will be increased number of macrophages, granulation tissue and ultimately fibrous tissue formation. Similar changes may also be seen with lymphadenopathy due to Actinomyces. In addition, sulfur granules that are large bacterial colonies should be evident. In lymphadenopathy due to Treponema pallidum there occurs follicular hyperplasia with interfollicular hyperplasia. Vessels are increased with features of vasculitis. Granulomas may or may not be present.

8. D

The broad categories of granulomatous lymphadenopathy are:

1. Infections (viral, bacterial, fungal, mycobacterial)
2. Systemic (sarcoidosis, rheumatoid arthritis, vasculitis)
3. In association with tumors (lymphomas, carcinomas, melanomas)
4. Foreign body
5. Immunodeficiency states

9. C

Kikuchi-Fujimoto disease is seen in Asian individuals especially in Japanese people. It is a rare disease, typically self-limiting, but with a small recurrence rate (3–4%). The etiology is not clear, although infective agents have been implicated. It is seen up to four times more often in females. Histology demonstrates necrotic areas in the paracortex with presence of karyorrhectic debris. The necrotic areas contain eosinophilic fibrinoid deposits. The necrotic areas are surrounded by numerous histiocytes. Neutrophils are absent. The disease is also known as necrotizing histiocytic lymphadenitis.

In typical cases of progressive transformation of germinal centers (PTGC) large lymphoid nodules are seen in a background of follicular hyperplasia. The large nodules are the progressively transformed germinal centers. It is thought that the cells of the mantle zone infiltrate and disrupt the germinal center. Tingible body macrophages are not seen. PTGC is considered to be a reactive process. It is, however, seen in association with nodular lymphocyte predominant Hodgkin lymphoma.

10. A

Kimura disease like Kikuchi disease is seen more often in the Asian population. The etiology is not known. This is a chronic inflammatory disorder of the subcutaneous tissue and affects regional lymph nodes. The cervical area is the most common site to be involved. Histology of the affected lymph nodes demonstrates follicular hyperplasia, eosinophilia with eosinophilic microabscesses and infiltration of the germinal centers. Increase in vessels may also be seen. Warthin Finkeldey giant cells may also be present.

11. D

Regressive changes in germinal centers is characterized by presence of small compact B-cell nodules where the germinal center B-cells are lost. Thus, the nodules consist of stromal elements. These findings can be seen in a variety of conditions including Castleman disease (hyaline vascular variant), HIV/AIDS, syphilis and post-chemotherapy and postradiation therapy.

12. B

Dermatopathic lymphadenitis is seen in lymph nodes draining areas of skin where there is inflammation or infection. Langerhans cells which are present in the skin migrate to the regional lymph nodes. T-cell hyperplasia with paracortical expansion is seen. Macrophages with brown pigment are present. The pigment is typically melanin.

Kawasaki disease is also known as mucocutaneous lymph node syndrome. This condition is seen more often in Japanese populations, affecting mostly children. There occurs expansion of the interfollicular areas with loss of normal architecture. Areas of necrosis with the presence of neutrophils and nuclear debris are seen.

13. D

Rosai Dorfman is also known as sinus histiocytosis with massive lymphadenopathy. It typically presents as bilateral painless cervical lymphadenopathy. The disease typically resolves spontaneously.

Histology shows dilatation of the sinuses with large foamy macrophages. They have round vesicular nuclei with nucleoli. Emperipolesis which is presence of intact lymphocytes within macrophages without their destruction is seen. Eosinophils are not prominent. The macrophages are positive for S100 and CD68, but are negative for CD1a.

14. A

Lymph nodes affected by Langerhans cell histiocytosis demonstrate sinusoidal dilatation by Langerhans cells. Langerhans cells have irregular nuclei with linear nuclear grooves. Eosinophils and multinucleated giant cells are seen. Langerhans cells are positive for S100, CD68 and CD1a.

15. A

Castleman disease (also known as anigofollicular hyperplasia) is broadly divided into two categories, localized and systemic (also known as multicentric). The types of localized disease include hyaline vascular variant and plasma cell variant.

The mediastinum is a common site of involvement. Involved areas demonstrate follicular hyperplasia. The follicles may show two or more germinal centers. The germinal centers are depleted of small lymphocytes. They are occupied by follicular dendritic cells. Hyaline deposits are found within the germinal centers. The mantle zone is expanded and often the mantle zone is composed of concentric rings. Sclerotic blood vessels are found to be radially penetrating the follicles. In the interfollicular areas there are increased blood vessels with plasma cells and lymphocytes, immunoblasts and eosinophils.

16. B

The exact etiology of Castleman disease remains unclear. However, there is an association with HHV-8 infection. Castleman disease may predispose to a variety of neoplasms including follicular dendritic cell sarcoma and malignant lymphoma.

Hematopoietic Neoplasms

Myeloid and Precursor Lymphoid Neoplasms: Questions 1–56

1. A 50-year-old man presents with fatigue and easy bruising. A complete blood count and peripheral blood smear shows leukocytosis with 56% circulating blasts. The patient has no previous history of myeloid neoplasm or treatment with chemotherapy. Which of the following findings would definitively establish a diagnosis of acute myeloid leukemia?
   A. Presence of blasts with deeply basophilic and vacuolated cytoplasm
   B. Presence of Auer rods in the blasts
   C. Presence of small blasts with round nuclei, variably dispersed chromatin, occasional nucleoli and scant amounts of basophilic cytoplasm
   D. Presence of large blasts with round nuclei, dispersed chromatin, prominent nucleoli and abundant basophilic cytoplasm

2. Which of the following findings would be most useful for establishing myeloid lineage in acute leukemia?
   A. Expression of CD13 by the blasts
   B. Expression of CD33 by the blasts
   C. Expression of myeloperoxidase by the blasts
   D. Expression of cytoplasmic CD3 by the blasts

3. Which of the following cell types would *not* be expected to express MPO?
   A. Myeloblasts
   B. Promyelocytes
   C. Monoblasts
   D. Promonocytes

4. Which of the following is *not* considered a "blast equivalent"?
   A. Atypical promyelocytes
   B. Atypical monocytes
   C. Promonocytes
   D. Monoblasts

5. Detection of which of the following molecular genetic abnormalities is equivalent to a diagnosis of acute myeloid leukemia, regardless of blast count?
   A. t(8;21)(q22;q22)
   B. t(9;11)(p22;q23)
   C. t(6;9)(p23;q34)
   D. t(3;3)(q21;q26.2)

6. Which of the following findings would <u>not</u> be expected in a patient with acute myeloid leukemia with t(8;21)(q22;q22); *RUNX1-RUNX1T1*?
   A. Presence of less than 20% blasts in the peripheral blood
   B. Dysplastic changes in the myeloid population
   C. Expression of CD19 in blasts
   D. Presence of numerous Auer rods in the blasts

7. The presence of increased eosinophilic precursors with abnormally large, basophilic granules in the bone marrow of a patient with acute myeloid leukemia is suggestive of which of the following cytogenetic abnormalities?
   A. t(8;21)(q22;q22); *RUNX1-RUNX1T1*
   B. t(15;17) (q22;q12); *PML-RARA*
   C. t(6;9)(p23;q34); *DEK-NUP214*
   D. inv(16)(p13.1q22); *CBFB-MYH11*

8. Which of the following statements regarding the "core binding factor leukemias" is *not* correct?
   A. These cases have a bad prognosis
   B. These cases should undergo molecular genetic testing for detection of *KIT* mutation
   C. These cases may show monocytic differentiation
   D. These cases may present as myeloid sarcoma

9. Which of the following molecular genetic abnormalities results in the disruption of core binding factor-α?
   A. inv(16)(p13.1q22)
   B. t(16;16)(p13.1;q22)
   C. t(6;9)(p23;q34)
   D. t(8;21)(q22;q22)

10. Which of the following statements regarding acute promyelocytic leukemia with *PML-RARA* is the most correct?
    A. The disease shows a poor response to treatment
    B. The disease is almost always preceded by chronic myelogenous leukemia
    C. Patients are at high risk for the development of disseminated intravascular coagulation
    D. Most patients present in the seventh or eighth decade of life

11. Which of the following morphologic findings is most suggestive of acute promyelocytic leukemia with *PML-RARA*?
    A. Presence of numerous eosinophils
    B. Blasts with prominent "cup-shaped" nuclei
    C. Blasts containing a single, slender Auer rod in the cytoplasm
    D. Cells containing numerous azurophilic granules and irregular, folded nuclei

12. Which of the following antigens is *not* typically expressed in acute promyelocytic leukemia with *PML-RARA*?
    A. CD13
    B. CD33
    C. MPO
    D. HLA-DR

13. Which of the following statements regarding the "microgranular variant" of acute promyelocytic leukemia with *PML-RARA* (APL) is the most correct?
    A. This variant often presents with a lower white blood cell count than typical APL
    B. The blasts contain numerous Auer rods in the cytoplasm
    C. The blasts in this variant are more likely to express HLA-DR and CD34
    D. This variant is less likely to result in disseminated intravascular coagulation

14. On which chromosome is the retinoic acid receptor α gene located?
    A. 15q22
    B. 17q12
    C. 17q11.2
    D. 11q13

15. A 50-year-old patient with a diagnosis of acute promyelocytic leukemia with *PML-RARA* undergoes bone marrow aspiration and biopsy after approximately two weeks of therapy. Which of the following statements is most correct?
    A. The presence of atypical promyelocytes in the bone marrow is indicative of treatment resistance and a poor prognosis
    B. Detection of *PML-RARA* fusion transcripts by RT-PCR would indicate a high risk of relapse
    C. Detection of *PML-RARA* fusion transcripts by RT-PCR would indicate a good prognosis
    D. The presence of atypical promyelocytes in the bone marrow would not affect prognosis

16. The presence of a *FLT3-ITD* mutation in acute promyelocytic leukemia with *PML-RARA* is associated with which of the following?
    A. Microgranular variant of disease
    B. Lower WBC count at presentation
    C. Resistance to all-*trans*-retinoic acid (ATRA)
    D. Increased sensitivity to all-*trans*-retinoic acid (ATRA)

17. Which of the following would be expected in acute promyelocytic leukemia with t(11;17)(q23;q12); *ZBTB16-RARA*?
    A. Increased sensitivity to all-*trans*-retinoic acid (ATRA)
    B. Increased sensitivity to arsenic trioxide
    C. Resistance to all-*trans*-retinoic acid (ATRA)
    D. No effect on response to treatment

18. Which of the following findings would *not* be expected in the blast population of acute myeloid leukemia with monocytic differentiation?
    A. Expression of CD14
    B. Expression of CD34
    C. Expression of CD64
    D. Expression of CD4

19. Which of the following is *not* associated with monocytic differentiation in acute myeloid leukemia?
    A. Disseminated intravascular coagulation
    B. Gingival involvement
    C. Central nervous system involvement
    D. Bone marrow fibrosis

20. Which of the following findings are *not* associated with translocations of the *MLL* (*KMT2A*)gene?
    A. Mixed phenotype acute leukemia
    B. Acute lymphoblastic leukemia
    C. History of previous treatment with etoposide
    D. History of Down's syndrome

21. Which of the following types of acute myeloid leukemia is *not* associated with multilineage dysplasia?
    A. Acute myeloid leukemia with *PML-RARA*
    B. Acute myeloid leukemia with t(8;21) (q22;q22); *RUNX1-RUNX1T1*
    C. Acute myeloid leukemia with t(6;9)(p23;q34); *DEK-NUP214*
    D. Acute myeloid leukemia with inv(3) (q21q26.2); *GATA2, MECOM*

22. Which of the following findings is *not* expected in acute myeloid leukemia with t(6;9)(p23;q34); *DEK-NUP214*?
    A. Thrombocytosis
    B. Basophilia
    C. Multilineage dysplasia
    D. Pancytopenia

23. Which of the following findings is *not* expected in acute myeloid leukemia with inv(3)(q21q26.2) or t(3;3)(q21;q26.2); *GATA2, MECOM*?
    A. Thrombocytosis
    B. Basophilia
    C. Multilineage dysplasia
    D. Increased megakaryocytes

24. Acute myeloid leukemia with t(1;22) (p13.3;q13.1); *RBM15-MKL1* is most likely to present in which of the following patients?
    A. A 5-year-old girl with Down's syndrome
    B. A 5-month-old girl without Down's syndrome
    C. A 5-month-old boy with Down's syndrome
    D. A 15-year-old girl with Down's syndrome

25. Which of the following is the strongest predictor of response to therapy in acute myeloid leukemia?
    A. Percentage of blasts in the peripheral blood
    B. Immunophenotype of the leukemic blasts
    C. Percentage of blasts in the bone marrow
    D. Karyotype of the leukemic blasts

26. Which of the following molecular genetic abnormalities would be most likely to impart a poor prognosis in a patient with acute myeloid leukemia?
    A. t(8;21)(q22;q22; *RUNX1-RUNX1T1*)
    B. t(16;16)(p13.1;q22); *CBFB-MYH11*
    C. 46, XY
    D. del(5q)

27. Which of the following cytogenetic findings is most commonly seen in the leukemic cells of patients with acute myeloid leukemia?
    A. t(8;21)(q22;q22); *RUNX1-RUNX1T1*
    B. Normal karyotype
    C. Complex karyotype
    D. t(15;17)(q22;q12);*PML-RARA*

28. A mutation in which of the following genes would be considered a "Class I" mutation in acute myeloid leukemia?
    A. *CEBPA*
    B. *MLL* (*KMT2A*)
    C. *FLT3*
    D. *NPM1*

29. All of the following are causes of blasts in the peripheral blood except:
    A. Myelodysplastic syndrome
    B. Chronic myeloid leukemia, *BCR-ABL1*+
    C. Chronic lymphocytic leukemia
    D. Sepsis

30. Chloroacetate esterase will stain all of the following cells except:
    A. Neutrophils
    B. Myeloblasts
    C. Mast cells
    D. Neoplastic eosinophils

31. Regarding acute promyelocytic leukemia:
    A. There are two distinct subtypes, classical and microgranular. The treatment of these two subtypes is distinctly different.
    B. The total WBC count in the microgranular variant is typically very high
    C. The leukemic cells typically lack CD117
    D. Prognosis for APL is poor due to high incidence of disseminated intravascular coagulation (DIC)

32. A newly diagnosed case of acute myeloid leukemia demonstrates positivity of blasts by flow cytometry for CD19 in addition to CD34, MPO, CD13 and HLA-DR. The most likely cytogenetic abnormality associated with this immunophenotype is:
    A. t(9;22)
    B. t(8;21)
    C. t(16;16)
    D. t(15;17)

33. A newly diagnosed case of acute myeloid leukemia demonstrates presence of blasts with "cup-like" nuclear invaginations. The most likely molecular association is:
    A. *BCR-ABL1*
    B. Mutated *JAK2*
    C. Mutated *NPM1*
    D. Mutated *CEBPA*

34. Which of the following statements, regarding acute lymphoblastic leukemia/lymphoma is false?
    A. It is the most common childhood malignancy
    B. Acute lymphoblastic leukemia and acute lymphoblastic lymphoma are clinically and biologically equivalent
    C. The majority of acute lymphoblastic leukemia cases are of B-cell origin
    D. The majority of acute lymphoblastic leukemia cases are of T-cell origin

35. Which of the following is an unfavorable factor for a child with B-lymphoblastic leukemia/lymphoma?
    A. Being six years of age
    B. Presence of t(12;21)(p13.2;q22.1); *ETV6-RUNX1*

C. Presence of *MLL* (*KMT2A*) gene rearrangement
D. Lack of central nervous system involvement at presentation

36. Which of the following antigens is specific for B-lymphoblastic leukemia/lymphoma by flow cytometry?
    A. CD19
    B. CD10
    C. TdT
    D. None of the above

37. Which of the following flow cytometry findings would not be expected in B-lymphoblastic leukemia/lymphoma?
    A. Expression of CD19
    B. Expression of CD20
    C. Expression of CD15
    D. Expression of surface Kappa light chain

38. A 70-year-old man presents with pancytopenia for six months. A bone marrow is performed and shows dysplasia in the granulocyte, erythrocyte and megakaryocyte lineages. The blast count in the peripheral blood is less than 1% and the blast count in the bone marrow is less than 5%. The best diagnosis is:
    A. Myelodysplastic syndrome with excess blasts-1
    B. Myelodysplastic syndrome with excess blasts-2
    C. Myelodysplastic syndrome with multilineage dysplasia
    D. Acute myeloid leukemia with myelodysplasia-related changes

39. All of the following are features of myelodysplastic syndrome with isolated del(5q) except:
    A. Increased incidence in females
    B. Blast count >1% in the peripheral blood
    C. Good prognosis
    D. Increased platelet count

40. Which of the following statements regarding abnormal localization of immature precursors (ALIP) is true?
    A. ALIP is a term used to describe presence of immature myeloid cells located in the paratrabecular areas

B. ALIP is frequently seen in cases of B12/folate deficiency

C. ALIP is frequently seen in myelodysplastic syndrome and imparts a worsened prognosis

D. ALIP is frequently seen in myelodysplastic syndrome and imparts a good prognosis

41. A 70-year-old man presents with pancytopenia for six months. A bone marrow examination shows a hypercellular bone marrow but no significant dysplasia. Which of the following cytogenetic abnormalities would be considered presumptive evidence for a diagnosis of myelodysplastic syndrome?
    A. del(7q)
    B. –Y
    C. +8
    D. del(20q)

42. Which of the following is not a feature of myelodysplastic syndrome with ringed sideroblasts?
    A. >15% ring sideroblasts (as a percentage of all erythroid cells)in the bone marrow
    B. Anemia
    C. 2% blasts with Auer rods in the peripheral blood
    D. Presence of *SF3B1* mutation

43. Which of the following statements regarding t(9;22)(q34;q11.2); *BCR-ABL1* and its resultant fusion proteins is false?
    A. The fusion protein p210 is most frequently seen in chronic myeloid leukemia, *BCR-ABL1* positive
    B. The fusion protein p190 is most frequently seen in Philadelphia chromosome-positive B-lymphoblastic leukemia/lymphoma
    C. The fusion protein p230 is associated with morphologic features that resemble chronic myelomonocytic leukemia
    D. The fusion protein p230 is associated with increased neutrophilic maturation in chronic myeloid leukemia

44. All of the following are features of accelerated phase of chronic myeloid leukemia, *BCR-ABL1* positive, except:
    A. Presence of a second Philadelphia chromosome
    B. Presence of 20% blasts in the peripheral blood

C. Presence of 20% basophils in the peripheral blood

D. Persistent thrombocytosis (>1000 x 10^9/L), unresponsive to therapy

45. All of the following are characteristic features of chronic myeloid leukemia, *BCR-ABL1* positive in chronic phase except:
    A. Small hypolobated megakaryocytes in the bone marrow
    B. Increased basophils in the peripheral blood and bone marrow
    C. Mild to moderate dysplasia in granulocytic precursors
    D. Presence of pseudo-Gaucher cells in the bone marrow

46. The highest incidence of *JAK2* mutation is seen in:
    A. Polycythemia vera
    B. Primary myelofibrosis
    C. Essential thrombocythemia
    D. Chronic myeloid leukemia, *BCR-ABL1* positive

47. All of the following abnormalities may be seen in primary myelofibrosis except:
    A. *JAK2* mutation
    B. *BCR-ABL1* fusion
    C. *CALR* mutation
    D. *MPL* mutation

48. All of the following are expected in the overt fibrotic phase of primary myelofibrosis except:
    A. Leukoerythroblastosis with prominent "tear-drop"-shaped red blood cells in the peripheral blood
    B. Intrasinusoidal hematopoiesis in the bone marrow
    C. Dyserythropoiesis
    D. Increased atypical megakaryocytes of variable size

49. Neoplastic mast cells are positive for:
    A. CD20
    B. CD3
    C. CD25
    D. CD117

50. Features expected in a case of atypical chronic myeloid leukemia include:
    A. Dysplasia in the granulocytic lineage

B. Presence of Philadelphia chromosome

C. Monocytosis

D. Basophilia

51. Which of the following is associated with marked peripheral blood eosinophilia?

A. B lymphoblastic leukemia/lymphoma with t(9;22)(q34.1;q11.2); *BCR-ABL1*

B. B lymphoblastic leukemia/lymphoma with t(v;11q23);*KMT2A* rearranged

C. B lymphoblastic leukemia/lymphoma with t(5;14)(q31;q32); *IL3-IGH*

D. B lymphoblastic leukemia/lymphoma with t(12;21)(p13;q22); *ETV6-RUNX1*

52. Which of the following is most likely to be seen in an infant?

A. B lymphoblastic leukemia/lymphoma with t(9;22)(q34.1;q11.2); *BCR-ABL1*

B. B lymphoblastic leukemia/lymphoma with t(v;11q23);*KMT2A* rearranged

C. B lymphoblastic leukemia/lymphoma with t(5;14)(q31;q32); *IL3-IGH*

D. B lymphoblastic leukemia/lymphoma with t(12;21)(p13;q22); *ETV6-RUNX1*

53. Which of the following has been definitively associated with a good prognosis?

A. B lymphoblastic leukemia/lymphoma with t(9;22)(q34.1;q11.2); *BCR-ABL1*

B. B lymphoblastic leukemia/lymphoma with t(v;11q23);*KMT2A* rearranged

C. B lymphoblastic leukemia/lymphoma with t(5;14)(q31;q32); *IL3-IGH*

D. B lymphoblastic leukemia/lymphoma with t(12;21)(p13;q22); *ETV6-RUNX1*

54. Which of the following statements regarding B lymphoblastic leukemia/lymphoma with t(9;22)(q34.1;q11.2); *BCR-ABL1* is false?

A. It is more frequently seen in children than in adults

B. It is more frequently seen in adults than in children

C. It is associated with a poor prognosis

D. It is associated with the p190 fusion transcript

55. Detection of which of the following antigens by flow cytometry is diagnostic of T-cell differentiation in acute lymphoblastic leukemia?

A. CD1a

B. Cytoplasmic CD22

C. Cytoplasmic CD3

D. Surface CD4

56. A bone marrow shows sheets of immature-appearing cells with the following immunophenotype: CD1a(-), cCD3(+), CD5(dim +), CD7 (+), CD13(+), CD33(+), CD34 (+), CD117(+), MPO(-), TdT(+). Which of the following is the best diagnosis?

A. T-cell lymphoblastic leukemia/lymphoma

B. Mixed phenotype acute leukemia, T/myeloid

C. Acute myeloid leukemia with minimal differentiation

D. Early T-precursor acute lymphoblastic leukemia

Answers to Chapter 4

1. B	15. D	29. C	43. C
2. C	16. A	30. B	44. B
3. C	17. C	31. B	45. C
4. B	18. B	32. B	46. A
5. A	19. D	33. C	47. B
6. D	20. D	34. D	48. C
7. D	21. A	35. C	49. C
8. A	22. A	36. D	50. A
9. D	23. B	37. D	51. C
10. C	24. B	38. C	52. B
11. D	25. D	39. B	53. D
12. D	26. D	40. C	54. A
13. C	27. B	41. A	55. C
14. B	28. C	42. C	56. D

Answers to Chapter 4 (with Explanations)

1. B

   Acute myeloid leukemia (AML) refers to a group of heterogeneous diseases that result from the clonal proliferation of myeloblasts in the peripheral blood, bone marrow and/or extramedullary tissue (myeloid sarcoma). Diagnosis of AML requires the presence of at least 20% myeloblasts in the peripheral blood and/or bone marrow or the presence of myeloid sarcoma. Accurate diagnosis and classification of AML requires correlation of clinical, morphologic, immunophenotypic and molecular genetic data. However, the first step involves establishment of myeloid differentiation. Although the morphology of lymphoblasts and myeloblasts is somewhat distinct, morphology alone is not sufficiently specific to establish lineage. One of the few exceptions to this is the detection of Auer rods in the blasts. Auer rods result from the abnormal fusion of primary neutrophilic granules and lysomes into rod-shaped cytoplasmic inclusions. These inclusions have a distinct purple-red color (referred to as azurophilic) when stained with Romanowsky-type stains such as Wright-Giemsa.

2. C

   Myeloperoxidase (MPO) is a peroxidase enzyme stored in the cytoplasmic granules of neutrophils and other myeloid cells. Its main function is to produce hypochlorous acid (HOCL) during the respiratory burst in neutrophils in order to kill bacteria and other pathogens. Its detection in blasts, either by cytochemistry, immunohistochemistry and/or flow cytometry establishes myeloid lineage. However, lack of MPO expression alone *does not* exclude myeloid lineage. Expression of myeloid-related antigens such as CD13, CD15 and CD33 can occasionally be seen in lymphoblasts. Expression of cytoplasmic CD3 is useful in establishing T-cell lineage.

3. C

   Although the majority of myeloid cells express myeloperoxidase (MPO), certain cell types do not. As such, lack of MPO expression does not rule out myeloid lineage in all cases. Very early or minimally differentiated myeloblasts (such as those in acute myeloid leukemia with minimal differentiation, AKA "M0" in the French-American-British classification), monoblasts and megakaryoblasts show little or no expression of MPO. However, the presence of ≥20% of these cell types in the peripheral blood and/or bone marrow, would still be indicative of acute myeloid leukemia. Although monoblasts usually lack MPO expression, promonocytes, which are considered monoblast equivalents, frequently express MPO.

4. B

   The diagnosis of acute myeloid leukemia (AML) generally requires the detection of ≥ 20% blasts of myeloid lineage in the peripheral blood and/or bone marrow. However, certain cell types are considered to be "blast equivalents" and are counted as "blasts" in the differential. Such cells include the atypical promyelocytes seen in acute promyelocytic leukemia (APL), monoblasts, promonocytes, megakaryoblasts and erythroblasts (in rare cases of pure acute erythroid leukemia). Monoblasts and promonocytes, although morphologically distinct, are counted together, and their combined percentage is reported as one blast count. Of note, atypical monocytes, often seen in diseases such as chronic myelomonocytic leukemia (CMML), are *not* considered to be blast equivalents. As such, distinguishing between monoblasts, promonocytes and atypical monocytes is a necessary, though admittedly difficult, part of the bone marrow and/or peripheral blood differential.

5. A

   There are several types of acute myeloid leukemia (AML) with defined recurrent cytogenetic abnormalities. However, a subset of recurrent cytogenetic abnormalities is considered to be diagnostic of AML regardless of blast count. As such, a diagnosis of AML can be made even if percentage of blasts in the peripheral blood and/or bone marrow is less than 20% when any of the following abnormalities is detected:

- t(8;21)(q22;q22); *RUNX1-RUNX1T1*
- inv(16) (p13.1q22), or t(16;16)(p13.1;q22); *CBFB-MYH11*
- t(15;17) (q22;q12); *PML-RARA*

6. D

The blasts of acute myeloid leukemia with t(8;21) (q22;q22); *RUNX1-RUNX1T1* may contain numerous "salmon-pink" granules, and prominent perinuclear "hofs." Auer rods are occasionally found in the blasts; however, they usually appear as a single long and slender rod with tapered ends; the presence of numerous overlapping Auer rods should raise the possibility of acute promyelocytic leukemia. Examination of the bone marrow may show dysplastic changes in the developing myeloid population; however, these features should *not* prompt a diagnosis of acute myeloid leukemia with myelodysplasia-related changes (AML-MRC). Increased eosinophilic precursors may also be noted in the bone marrow; however, dysplastic eosinophils, as seen in acute myeloid leukemia with inv(16)(p13.1q22) or t(16;16) (p13.1;q22), are *not* seen in this disease. The blast cells show an immunophenotype consistent with myeloid lineage (including expression of CD13, CD33 and myeloperoxidase) but often show aberrant expression of antigens normally associated with B-lymphocytes including CD19, PAX-5 and cytoplasmic CD79a. Finally, rare cases of "hypoproliferative" disease or cases initially presenting as myeloid sarcoma may be encountered. The peripheral blood in such cases may show leukopenia and < 20% blasts; however, detection of t(8;21) will allow for the diagnosis of acute myeloid leukemia.

7. D

Both inv(16)(p13.1q22) and t(16;16)(p13.1;q22) result in fusion of the *CBFB* gene at 16q22 to the *MYH11* gene at 16p13.1. Evaluation of the bone marrow in patients with acute myeloid leukemia and either of these abnormalities often shows variable numbers of immature eosinophil precursors (often in the promyelocyte or myelocyte stage of maturation). The granules present in these eosinophilic precursors frequently obscure the nucleus and are often large and basophilic. The presence of such "dysplastic" eosinophilic granules is highly suggestive of acute myeloid leukemia with either inv(16)(p13.1q22) or t(16;16)(p13.1;q22); *CBF-MYH11*.

8. A

Core binding factor (CBF) is a transcription factor that is necessary for normal hematopoiesis. Disruption of its function results in leukemogenesis. Acute myeloid leukemia with t(8;21)(q22;q22) and acute myeloid leukemia with inv(16) (p13.1q22) or t(16;16)(p13.1;q22) are generally referred to as the "core binding factor leukemias" because they both result in disruption of CBF function. The t(8;21)(q22;q22) results in fusion of the *RUNX1* gene (also known as core binding factor-α and *AML1*) with the *RUNX1T1* gene (also known as ETO). AML with inv(16)(p13.1q22) or t(16;16) (p13.1;q22) involves core binding factor-β and the *MYH11* gene. Therefore, t(8;21)(q22;q22) disrupts the α-subunit of CBF and inv(16)(p13.1q22) or t(16;16)(p13.1;q22) disrupts the β-subunit of CBF. As a result, both types of leukemia show similar clinicopathologic features. The core binding factor leukemias have an overall good response to chemotherapy and a good prognosis. However, the presence of a concurrent mutation in the *KIT* gene is found in approximately 20–25% of cases and is associated with a worsened prognosis. As such, all cases of core binding factor leukemia should undergo testing for this mutation. The core binding factor leukemias have increased propensity for monocytic differentiation and extramedullary involvement (myeloid sarcoma). Myeloid sarcoma may precede, or appear concurrently with, bone marrow involvement or be the first manifestation of relapse.

9. D

Acute myeloid leukemia with t(8;21)(q22;q22); *RUNX1-RUNX1T1* disrupts the α-subunit of core binding factor, while acute myeloid leukemia with inv(16)(p13.1q22) or t(16;16)(p13.1;q22); *CBFB-MYH11* disrupts the β-subunit of core binding factor.

10. C

Rare cases of chronic myeloid leukemia (CML) that go into "blast phase" may transform into acute promyelocytic leukemia with *PML-RARA* (APL)(formally acute promyelocytic leukemia with t(15;17)(q22;q12); *PML-RARA*); however, the disease most often presents de-novo and shows an abrupt onset. It is most common in children and young adults, with most cases presenting before the sixth decade of life. APL shows a good response to anthracycline-based chemotherapy, arsenic trioxide and all-*trans*-retinoic acid (ATRA). However, especially prior to treatment, patients are at high risk for development of life-threating disseminated intravascular coagulation (DIC). As such, close observation of coagulation studies (PT, PTT, fibrinogen and D-Dimer) is essential in the early phase of the disease.

11. D

Actual myeloblasts are rare in acute promyelocytic leukemia with *PML-RARA* (formally acute promyelocytic leukemia with t(15;17)(q22;q12); *PML-RARA*)The dominant cell type, which is considered a "blast equivalent," is the atypical promyelocyte. These cells are intermediate to large in size and contain numerous large granules in the cytoplasm. The granules are frequently azurophilic and often obscure the nucleus. The nuclei are highly irregular and may have a bilobed appearance that is referred to as "butterfly wing" or "apple-core" morphology. However, the most characteristic finding is the presence of numerous Auer rods in the cytoplasm. The Auer rods are short and thick, as opposed to the long and slender forms seen in acute myeloid leukemia with t(8;21)(q22;q22); *RUNX1-RUNX1T1*. They are also present in large numbers and often coalesce into bundles resembling a pile of firewood. Cytochemical staining with myeloperoxidase (MPO) will be strongly positive in the granules and Auer rods and will characteristically obscure visualization of the nucleus.

12. D

The neoplastic cells of acute promyelocytic leukemia with *PML-RARA* (APL) (formally acute promyelocytic leukemia with t(15;17)(q22;q12); *PML-RARA*) are characterized by low or absent expression of HLA-DR and CD34. They also lack expression of the leukocyte integrins CD11a, CD11b and CD18. Although CD15 expression is commonly seen in promyelocytes, the atypical promyelocytes of APL are usually negative for CD15. The neoplastic cells express CD13, CD33 (brightly), CD64, CD117 and myeloperoxidase (MPO). A subset of cases shows aberrant expression of CD56, which is associated with a worsened prognosis. Owing to the marked granularity of the cytoplasm, the neoplastic cells characteristically also show high side scatter when examined by flow cytometry.

13. C

The "microgranular variant" of acute promyelocytic leukemia with *PML-RARA* (formally acute promyelocytic leukemia with t(15;17)(q22;q12); *PML-RARA*) shows similar clinicopathologic features to the "typical" or "hypergranular" variant, including an acute onset, good response to treatment, high risk of disseminated intravascular coagulation, high side scatter on flow cytometry and strong expression of myeloperoxidase. However, the neoplastic cells in the microgranular variant are more likely to show dim expression of CD34 and HLA-DR. The neoplastic cells of both variants also have highly irregular, occasionally bilobed nuclei with "butterfly wing" or "apple-core" morphology. However, neoplastic cells in the microgranular variant show sparse granularity which allows for better visualization of the characteristic apple-core/butterfly wing shape of the nuclei. Occasional Auer rods are observed in the microgranular variant, but are not as abundant as in typical APL. In addition, the microgranular variant generally presents with a higher WBC count and a higher percentage of circulating atypical promyelocytes than typical APL.

14. B

The retinoic acid receptor α gene (*RARA*) is located on chromosome 17 band q12. The t(15;17)(q22;q12) results in the fusion of the *RARA* gene with the promyelocytic leukemia gene (*PML*) on chromosome 15, band q22, resulting in a *PML-RARA* fusion gene which blocks maturation of the cells past the promyelocyte stage. Treatment with all-*trans*-retinoic acid (ATRA) targets *RARA* and promotes differentiation of the neoplastic cells, whereas treatment with arsenic trioxide (ATO) targets *PML*, promoting maturation and apoptosis. Treatment with ATRA and ATO, often in combination with anthracycline-based therapy, is highly effective and is associated with high rates of complete remission.

15. **D**

It is possible to see atypical promyelocytes and detect *PML-RARA* transcripts by RT-PCR in the bone marrow for several weeks after initiation of treatment. This is thought to be due to the differentiation and apoptosis induced by the treatment, but is still incompletely understood. Nevertheless, these findings do not appear to indicate treatment resistance or impact prognosis. In contrast, detection of *PML-RARA* transcripts in a bone marrow from a patient who has completed induction therapy and achieved complete remission would be highly suggestive of impending relapse.

16. **A**

Mutations in the fms-related tyrosine kinase 3 gene (*FLT3*), located on chromosome 13q12, occur in a significant number of patients with acute promyelocytic leukemia with *PML-RARA* (formally acute promyelocytic leukemia with t(15;17)(q22;q12); *PML-RARA*). The majority of mutations are due to an internal tandem duplication (ITD) in the juxtamembrane region of the gene which results in constitutive activation. The presence of a *FLT3-ITD* mutation in patients with acute promyelocytic leukemia with *PML-RARA* is associated with a higher white blood cell count at diagnosis, microgranular variant of disease and involvement of the breakpoint region 3 (BCR3) region of the *PML* gene. The presence of this mutation is not known to effect response to all-*trans*-retinoic acid (ATRA) and its effect on prognosis remains unclear.

17. **C**

A subset of cases of acute promyelocytic leukemia has a translocation that results in the fusion of the retinoic acid receptor α gene (*RARA)* with a gene *other than* the promyelocytic leukemia gene (*PML*). Such cases are referred to as acute promyelocytic leukemia with variant *RARA* translocations. Although these cases show some clinicopathologic overlap with acute promyelocytic leukemia with *PML-RARA*, some variant translocations result in resistance to all-*trans*-retinoic acid (ATRA). Common variant partner genes include:

- *ZBTB16* gene at chromosome 11q23
- *NUMA1* gene at chromosome 11q13
- *NPM1* gene at chromosome 5q35
- *STAT5B* gene at chromosome 17q11.2

Acute promyelocytic leukemia with t(11;17)(q23;q12); *ZBTB16-RARA* has distinctive morphologic features. Recognition of this variant translocation is crucial, as this variant is resistant to ATRA. The neoplastic cells have round nuclei rather than the irregular, "apple-core" nuclei that are usually encountered. The cytoplasm is highly granular and strongly positive for myeloperoxidase, but Auer rods are usually absent. In addition, neutrophils with "pelgeroid" morphology (resembling the morphology of neutrophils seen in Pelger-Huet anomaly) are associated with this variant translocation and are a useful diagnostic clue. Fusion with the *STAT5B* gene on 17q11.2 is also associated with resistance to ATRA. Fusion with *NUMA1* or *NPM1* is *not* associated with ATRA resistance.

18. **B**

Acute myeloid leukemia (AML) with monocytic differentiation (AML-M4 and AML-M5 in the French-American-British Classification) contains variable amounts of monoblasts, promonocytes and monocytes. As such, the blasts express multiple monocytic antigens such as CD4, CD14, CD36 and CD64. They show aberrant expression of CD117 and, occasionally, CD56. Monoblasts are frequently negative for myeloperoxidase (MPO) while promonocytes may show MPO expression. Although CD34 is often a useful antigen for detection of blasts, it is important to note that cases of AML with monocytic differentiation may show no or very little expression of CD34.

19. **D**

There are numerous subtypes of acute myeloid leukemia that have an increased tendency toward monocytic differentiation including acute myeloid leukemia with t(8;21)(q22;q22); *RUNX1-RUNX1T1*, acute myeloid leukemia with inv(16)(p13.1q22) or t(16;16)(p13.1;q22); *CBFB-MYH11*, acute myeloid leukemia with t(9;11)(p22;q23); *MLLT3-KMT2A* (formally *MLLT3-MLL*), acute myeloid leukemia with mutated *NPM1* and others. Monocytic differentiation (which refers to the presence of variable amounts of monoblasts, promonocytes and monocytes) imparts certain characteristics that may complicate diagnosis including lack of CD34 expression and lack of myeloperoxidase expression. Cytochemical expression of nonspecific esterase in these cases is a useful diagnostic tool but is not available in all laboratories. However, detection of monocytic differentiation is crucial, especially in the initial, pretreatment phase of care. Patients with acute myeloid leukemia with monocytic differentiation are at increased risk of disseminated intravascular coagulation, leukostasis and extramedullary involvement of locations such as the skin, gingiva, heart and central nervous system. Ironically, many of the subtypes of acute myeloid leukemia which have a tendency towards monocytic differentiation have a relatively good or intermediate prognosis with treatment, but carry a significant risk of morbidity and mortality in the pre-treatment phase. Knowledge of and close monitoring for these potential complications is crucial in order to reduce the risk of mortality before initiation of treatment.

20. D

Translocations involving the *KMT2A* (formally *MLL)* gene on chromosome 11q23 can be seen in acute myeloid leukemia, acute lymphoblastic leukemia, therapy-related acute myeloid leukemia, acute myeloid leukemia with myelodysplasia-related changes, mixed phenotype acute leukemia and acute myeloid leukemia not otherwise specified. Acute myeloid leukemia in Down's syndrome is associated with several genetic abnormalities, but is not typically associated with translocation of the *MLL* (*KMT2A*)gene.

21. A

Many of the World Health Organization-defined "acute myeloid leukemias with recurrent genetic abnormalities" have the potential to display varying degrees of multilineage dysplasia. It is important to be aware of this possibility to avoid mistakenly labelling such cases as acute myeloid leukemia with myelodysplasia-related changes (AML-MRC). The following recurrent genetic abnormalities have the potential to display multilineage dysplasia:

- Acute myeloid leukemia with t(8;21) (q22;q22); *RUNX1-RUNX1T1*
- Acute myeloid leukemia with inv(16) (p13.1q22) or t(16;16)(p13.1;q22); *CBFB-MYH11*

- Acute myeloid leukemia with t(6;9)(p23;q34); *DEK-NUP214*
- Acute myeloid leukemia with inv(3) (q21q26.2); *GATA2, MECOM* (formally *RPN1-EVI1*)

Detection of any of these genetic abnormalities takes precedence over the presence of multilineage dysplasia, and these cases should not be classified as AML-MRC. This is mainly because some cases, such as acute myeloid leukemia with t(8;21) (q22;q22); *RUNX1-RUNX1T1* and acute myeloid leukemia with inv(16)(p13.1q22) or t(16;16) (p13.1;q22); *CBFB-MYH11* have a good response to treatment and good prognosis, as opposed to the bad prognosis seen in AML-MRC. Acute myeloid leukemia with t(6;9)(p23;q34); *DEK-NUP214* and acute myeloid leukemia with inv(3) (q21q26.2); *GATA2, MECOM* have an overall bad prognosis but should be still be classified separately from AML-MRC.

22. A

Acute myeloid leukemia with t(6;9)(p23;q34); *DEK-NUP214* most frequently occurs in children and young adults and often presents with pancytopenia. In addition, the median white blood cell count at presentation is lower than other types of AML. Furthermore, the bone marrow frequently shows multilineage dysplasia. As such, there is a potential for these cases to be misclassified as acute myeloid leukemia with myelodysplasia-related changes. However, the presence of the t(6;9) takes precedence over the presence of multilineage dysplasia. A useful clue to the diagnosis is the presence of peripheral blood and bone marrow basophilia, which is present in approximately 50% of cases. The overall prognosis for these cases is poor.

23. B

Acute myeloid leukemia with inv(3)(q21q26.2) or t(3;3)(q21;q26.2); *GATA2, MECOM* (formally *RPN1-EVI1*)is a rare subtype of AML that may present de-novo or after a history of myelodysplastic syndrome (MDS). These cases often show multilineage dysplasia and have a poor prognosis. Patients may present with thrombocytosis and the peripheral blood may have large, hypogranular platelets. Occasionally, circulating megakaryocyte nuclei may be found in the peripheral blood.

In addition, megakaryocytes may be increased and may show monolobated or bilobed nuclei.

24. B

Acute myeloid leukemia with t(1;22)(p13.3;q13.1); *RBM15-MKL1* occurs almost exclusively in infants, and appears to be more common in females. The disease results from the proliferation of megakaryoblasts and commonly presents as an extramedullary mass with or without marrow involvement. These cases are classified separately from cases of myeloid leukemia associated with Down syndrome, which also show megakaryocytic differentiation. Both types of disease are present in children; however, myeloid leukemia associated with Down syndrome can present "later" in life (within the first five years of life) and frequently shows multilineage dysplasia, a feature which is typically absent in acute myeloid leukemia with t(1;22)(p13;q13); *RBM15-MKL1*. Correlation with clinical history, physical examination and karyotype to assess for the presence of trisomy 21 can aid in the differentiation between these two subtypes of disease.

25. D

Many factors affect the prognosis of patients with acute myeloid leukemia. Patient-related factors, such as age, presence of co-morbidities and performance status strongly influence prognosis and are especially important in predicting therapy-related mortality (i.e. death resulting from complications of cytotoxic therapy such as infection, etc.). Leukemia-related factors are imparted by the specific leukemic clone or clones proliferating in the patient. These factors include morphology, immunophenotype, blast count, white blood cell count and karyotype and are especially important in predicting response to conventional therapy. These factors can be used to determine if a patient would benefit from more intensive regimens, use of investigational agents and so on. Furthermore, these factors can be specifically targeted in therapeutic regimens (e.g. use of all-trans-retinoid acid in acute promyelocytic leukemia with t(15;17); *PML-RARA*). Of all of the leukemia-related factors, the karyotype of the leukemic cells is the strongest predictor of response to therapy and survival. As such, conventional cytogenetic analysis is mandatory in all cases of acute myeloid leukemia.

26. D

It is well established that the karyotype of the leukemic cells is the strongest predictor of response to therapy and survival. However, knowledge of the numerous potential cytogenetic and molecular genetic abnormalities that may occur in the leukemic cells of acute myeloid leukemia, their interactions with each other and their effect on prognosis is expanding rapidly. In addition, much information has been gained about the prognostic effect of mutations in the nucleophosmin gene 1 (*NPM1*), internal tandem duplications in the fms-like tyrosine kinase 3 gene (*FLT3-ITD*) and bi-allelic mutations of the CCAAT enhancer binding protein α gene (*CEBPA*). Mutations in these genes allow for better prognostic stratification of patients whose leukemic cells show a normal karyotype. Although full characterization of the "molecular genetic landscape" in acute myeloid leukemia is still under investigation, certain abnormalities can be grouped into favorable, intermediate and adverse risk groups:

Favorable:

- t(8;21)(q22;q22); *RUNX1-RUNX1T1*
- inv(16)(p13.1q22) or t(16;16)(p13.1;q22); *CBFB-MYH11*
- t(15;17)(q22;q12);*PML-RARA*
- Normal karyotype with mutated *NPM1* and without *FLT3-ITD*
- Normal karyotype with bi-allelic mutated *CEBPA*

Intermediate:

- Normal karyotype
- Normal karyotype with mutated *NPM1* and *FLT3-ITD*
- Normal karyotype with wild-type *NPM1* and *FLT3-ITD*
- t(9;11)(p22;q23); *MLLT3-KMT2A* (formally *MLL*)

Adverse:

- inv(3)(q21q26.2) or t(3;3)(q21;q26.2); *GATA2, MECOM* (formally *RPN1-EVI1*)
- t(6;9)(p23;q34); *DEK-NUP214*
- t(v;11)(v;q23); *KMT2A* (formally *MLL*) rearranged
- -5 or del(5q)
- -7
- Complex karyotype (≥3 chromosomal abnormalities)

27. B

Although the karyotype of the leukemic cells in acute myeloid leukemia is the strongest predictor of response to therapy and survival, the most frequently encountered leukemic karyotype (45–55% of cases) is a normal karyotype. Such cases are often referred to as "Normal Karyotype AML" or "Cytogenetically Normal AML" and are categorized as having an intermediate prognosis. As would be expected, these cases show highly variable survival rates and a heterogeneous response to therapy. The recognition of the prognostic impact of certain genetic mutations (especially in genes such as *NPM1*, *FLT3* and *CEBPA*) in normal karyotype AML has allowed for better risk stratification in these patients. As such, testing for mutations in *NPM1*, *FLT3* and *CEBPA* should be considered mandatory in cases of normal karyotype AML.

28. C

The impact of various genetic mutations on leukemogenesis and prognosis is an area of ongoing investigation. The importance of these mutated genes lies in their potential effect on leukemogenesis (cellular proliferation, cellular maturation, epigenetic modification, etc.) as well as the effect of their interaction with other types of mutations. Certain mutation types may "work together" to initiate leukemogenesis, promote survival of leukemic clones and resist or survive standard chemotherapeutic regimens. In broad terms, these mutations can be divided into two "classes" or "types" which have the potential to interact with each other and promote the growth and survival of leukemic clones. "Class I" mutations promote proliferation and survival but do not affect differentiation. Class I mutations are likely later events in leukemogenesis, frequently involve receptor tyrosine kinases and strongly affect prognosis but do not define exclusive subtypes of AML. Class II mutations impair hematopoietic cell differentiation and apoptosis. These mutations appear to be initiating events in leukemogenesis and often define exclusive subtypes of AML. Examples of each are listed here:

- Class I Mutations
  - *FLT3-ITD*
  - *KIT*
  - *RAS*
  - *JAK2*

- Class II Mutations
  - *NPM1*
  - *CEBPA*
  - *KMT2A* (formally *MLL*)
  - *PML-RARA*
  - *RUNX1-RUNX1T1*
  - *CBFB-MYH11*

29. C

Blasts may be seen in the peripheral blood in a wide variety of situations. These include:

- Acute leukemia
- CML
- MDS
- Neupogen effect
- Neonates with an underlying reactive process
- Leukoerythroblastic blood picture (which can be seen in hemorrhage, hemolysis, or sepsis)
- Leukemoid reaction

Patients with chronic lymphocytic leukemia (CLL) do not undergo blast transformation. Individuals with CLL demonstrate lymphocytes with atypical morphology as well as a variable number of prolymphocytes. These are larger cells with abundant blue cytoplasm and nuclei with nucleoli. They are morphologically distinct from blasts.

30. B

Although cytochemical techniques have largely been replaced by immunohistochemistry and flow cytometry, they remain useful for detecting certain subsets of cells.

Chloroacetate esterase stains cells of the neutrophil lineage, mast cells, and shows positivity in the neoplastic eosinophils of acute myeloid leukemia with inv(16)(p13.1q22) or t(16;16)(p13.1;q22); *CBFB-MYH11*.

The detection of myeloperoxidase (MPO) in blasts by cytochemistry establishes myeloid lineage but a lack of cytochemical MPO expression does not rule out myeloid lineage. Myeloperoxidase (MPO) normally stains myeloblasts in a granular and Golgi distribution. However, the presence of numerous, strongly MPO-positive granules that obscure the nucleus should raise suspicion for a diagnosis of acute promyelocytic leukemia. Monoblasts usually lack MPO expression, but strongly express non-specific esterase (NSE).

Promonocytes (which are considered equivalent to monoblasts) are often NSE positive and may show weak expression of MPO.

31. B

There are two subtypes of acute promyelocytic leukemia (APL with *PML-RARA*). These are the classical and the microgranular subtypes. In the classical subtypes, abnormal promyelocytes with abundant granules are seen. Auer rods are easily visualized. In the microgranular variant the granules are not visible by light microscopy. The nuclei of these cells are abnormal. They have a bilobed appearance. The WBC count in the microgranular variant is typically very high. The incidence of disseminated intravascular coagulation (DIC) is high in APL. The treatment of both subtypes is the same and both subtypes have a good prognosis

32. B

The immunophenotype of acute myeloid leukemia with t(8;21)(q22;q22.1); *RUNX1-RUNX1T1* is characterized by aberrant expression of B-cell associated antigens such as CD19.

33. C

The presence of "cup-like" or "fish-mouth"-like nuclear indentations in the blasts of acute myeloid leukemia has been associated with mutations of the *NPM1* and *FLT-3* genes.

34. D

Acute lymphoblastic leukemia/lymphoma (ALL) is the most common childhood malignancy. Acute lymphoblastic leukemia (ALL) and acute lymphoblastic lymphoma (LBL) are biologically equivalent. Cases are designated as ALL when there is predominantly blood and bone marrow involvement (>25% lymphoblasts in the bone marrow) and are designated as LBL when there is predominantly extramedullary involvement with no or little blood/bone marrow involvement (<25% lymphoblasts in the bone marrow). The clinical and biologic differences between the two diseases appears to be minimal; however, the vast majority (80–85%) of ALL cases are of B-cell origin, while the vast majority of LBL cases are of T-cell origin In particular, LBL involvement of the mediastinum is almost always of T-cell origin. Clinical features include fever, bone pain/joint pain (especially in pediatric patients), organomegaly, pallor, fatigue, easy bleeding/bruising,

central nervous system involvement and testis involvement in males. Patients also frequently have severe anemia, thrombocytopenia, and neutropenia due to bone marrow involvement. The white blood cell count may be normal, decreased, or elevated.

35. C

B-lymphoblastic leukemia/lymphoma (B-ALL) has a high cure rate and favorable prognosis in children. However the prognosis is worse in adults, owing to the higher incidence of t(9;22)(q34.1;q11.2); *BCR-ABL1* (Philadelphia chromosome) in this subset of patients.

Favorable factors for B-ALL include:

- Age 2–10 years at diagnosis
- Rapid response to induction therapy (considered to be one of the most important prognostic factors)
- Lack of minimal residual disease after therapy
- WBC count less than 50,000/mm³ of blood at presentation
- Absence of central nervous system disease at diagnosis
- High hyperdiploidy (>50 chromosomes in neoplastic cells)
- Presence of t(12;21)(p13.2;q22.1); *ETV6-RUNX1*

Unfavorable factors for B-ALL include:

- > 10 years of age at diagnosis
- <1 year of age at diagnosis owing to frequent presence of *KMT2A* (formally *MLL*) gene rearrangement in this subset of patients
- Slow response to induction chemotherapy
- Presence of minimal residual disease after therapy
- High WBC count (>50,000/mm³) at diagnosis
- Presence of central nervous system involvement at diagnosis
- Hypodiploidy (<46 chromosomes in neoplastic cells)
- Presence of t(9;22)(q34.1;q11.2); *BCR-ABL1* (Philadelphia chromosome)
- Presence of *KMT2A* (formally *MLL*) gene rearrangement
- Presence of intrachromosomal amplification of one copy of chromosome 21 (iAMP21)

36. D

No single antigen can be used to reliably diagnose or exclude B-lymphoblastic leukemia/lymphoma (B-ALL). Flow cytometry is a powerful diagnostic technique because it allows for the simultaneous evaluation of *multiple* antigens in a cell population. In general, B-ALL is diagnosed by flow cytometry by the detection of (1)antigens associated with immaturity (such as CD34 and TdT) combined with (2) markers associated with B-cell lineage (such as CD10, CD19, cytoplasmic CD22 and CD79a), and (3) aberrant antigen expression (expression of antigens not normally seen in B-lymphocytes) and/or aberrant antigen expression patterns. These cells should be present in the traditional "blast gate" (dim/negative CD45 and low side scatter).

The following immunophenotypic findings are considered to be sufficient to assign B-cell lineage:

- Strong CD19 with *at least one* of the following: CD10 (strong), cytoplasmic CD22, CD79a,
- Weak CD19, with *at least two* of the following: CD10 (strong), cytoplasmic CD22, CD79a

Common antigens of immaturity include:

- CD34
- TdT
- HLA-DR (not a specific marker of immaturity; is also expressed by monocytes, mature B-cells, and activated T-cells)
- Lack of surface immunoglobulin expression
- Dim or negative CD45

Common aberrant antigen expression includes

- *Dim* expression of CD13 and CD33
- Expression of CD15 (often with lack of CD10 expression in cases with *KMT2A* [formally *MLL*] gene rearrangement)
- Expression of CD20
- Dim CD38 expression

37. D

Expression of B-lineage markers such as CD19, cytoplasmic CD22 and CD79a are commonly seen in B-lymphoblastic leukemia/lymphoma (B-ALL).

CD20 expression is associated with B-cell maturity but is seen in a subset of B-ALL cases (approximately 20–40%). The presence or absence of CD20 should always be reported because patients with CD20-positive B-ALL may benefit from the addition of rituximab (an anti-CD20 catalytic antibody) to their therapeutic regimen.

Aberrant expression of myeloid antigens such as CD13, CD14, CD15, CD33 and CD65 is seen in a subset of B-ALL. These antigens often show dim expression. CD15 is often expressed in patients with *KMT2A* (formally *MLL* gene rearrangement). Of note, very dim expression of myeloperoxidase can rarely be seen in B-ALL. Thus, the full immunophenotype of such cases should be examined in order to avoid an incorrect diagnosis of mixed phenotype acute leukemia.

In contrast, B-ALL should not show strong expression of surface light chains (Kappa and Lambda). The presence of surface light chain expression implies maturity and an alternative diagnosis such as Burkitt lymphoma, should be sought.

38. C

Myelodysplastic syndrome (MDS) is a clonal hematopoietic neoplasm characterized by the presence of *persistent* and *progressive* peripheral blood cytopenias, a hypercellular bone marrow, and the presence of dysplastic morphology in ≥10% of cells in one or more hematopoietic lineages.

There are many subtypes of MDS and they can be broadly grouped into "low-grade" and "high-grade" disease. Low grade MDS has a longer median survival and a lower rate of progression to acute myeloid leukemia than high grade disease.

The low-grade MDS subtypes have <1% blasts in the peripheral blood (PB) and <5% blasts in the bone marrow (BM). The blasts do not contain Auer rods. These cases are further subdivided by the number of dysplastic lineages present and the presence of ring sideroblasts. A unique subtype is defined by the isolated presence of deletion of chromosome 5q.:

- MDS with single lineage dysplasia
- MDS with ring sideroblasts (MDS-RS)
  - MDS-RS and single lineage dysplasia
  - MDS-RS and multilineage dysplasia
- MDS with multilineage dysplasia
- MDS with isolated del(5q)

The high grade MDS subtypes are further subdivided by the blast count:

- MDS with excess blasts-1(MDS-EB-1): 2–4% blasts in PB, 5–9% blasts in BM without Auer rods
- MDS with excess blasts-2 (MDS-EB-2): 5–19% blasts in PB, 10–19% blasts in BM. The presence of Auer rods (with any blast %) is automatically classified as MDS-EB-2.

Cases with ≥20% blasts in the PB or BM should be classified as acute myeloid leukemia with myelodysplasia-related changes.

Thus, in this case with dysplasia in all three lineages, <1% blast in the PB, and < 5% blasts in the BM, the best diagnosis is myelodysplastic syndrome with multilineage dysplasia (MDS-MLD). This entity was formally termed "refractory cytopenia with multilineage dysplasia (RCMD)".

39. B

Myelodysplastic syndrome with isolated deletion of chromosome 5q [MDS with isolated del(5q)] is a distinct subtype of MDS with unique clinicopathologic features and an excellent prognosis.

Unlike other types of MDS (which show a higher incidence in men), MDS with isolated del(5q) is more common in women. Patients present with anemia (usually macrocytic) and normal or increased platelet counts. The bone marrow is either normocellular or hypercellular and may show erythroid hypoplasia with no or only minimal dysplasia in the erythroid and myeloid lineages. In contrast, the megakaryocytes are usually increased and shows prominent monolobated nuclei. The peripheral blood has <1% blasts and the bone marrow has <5% blasts. Blasts cannot contain Auer rods. Ring sideroblasts may be observed. Cases with 1% blasts in the peripheral blood (measured on two separate occasions) should be classified as myelodysplastic syndrome unclassifiable (MDS-U). Cases with higher blast counts or Auer rods should be classified as myelodysplastic syndrome with excess blasts (MDS-EB).

Recently, it has been shown that the presence of one additional cytogenetic abnormality does not affect prognosis as long as the additional cytogenetic abnormality is not deletion of chromosome 7 or 7q. These cases may still be classified as MDS with isolated del(5q).

Interestingly, rare cases of MDS with isolated del(5q) and concurrent *JAK2 V617F* mutation have also been reported. The effect of this additional abnormality is not fully understood but reported cases seem to retain the good prognosis of MDS with isolated del(5q). These cases may still be classified as MDS with isolated del(5q) but the presence of *JAK2 V617F* should be reported.

40. C

Myeloid maturation typically occurs in the paratrabecular and perivascular regions of the bone marrow. Abnormal localization of immature precursors (ALIP) refers to the presence of clustered, immature myeloid cells in the central (nonparatrabecular) portion of the bone marrow. Three or more foci fulfil the criteria for ALIP. ALIP is often seen in high-grade myelodysplastic syndrome, such as myelodysplastic syndrome with excess blasts.

41. A

Cytogenetic abnormalities are seen in 50–60% of patients with myelodysplastic syndrome (MDS). Certain abnormalities are so closely associated with MDS that their detection can be considered presumptive evidence of MDS in the absence of significant dysplasia. However, a diagnosis of MDS should only be made if the patient also has significant and persistent (at least 6 months) cytopenias. These abnormalities include:

- -7 or del(7q)
- -5 or del(5q)
- +21 or -21
- -17, i(17q) or unbalanced translocations at 17p
- del(11q)
- del(9q)
- +6
- Del(12p) or unbalanced translocations at 12p
- -13 or del(13q)
- Any of the following translocations:
  ○ t(3;3)(q21q26)
  ○ t(3;21)(q26;q22)
  ○ inv3(q21q26)

○ t(1;7)(p11;p11)

○ t(2;11)(p21;q23)

○ t(11;16)(q23;p13)

○ t(6;9)(p23;q34)

○ t(2;11)(p21;q23)

Of the preceding, the most commonly seen abnormalities in MDS are -5/5q and -7/7q. The remaining abnormalities, especially the translocations, are infrequently seen.

The following abnormalities are frequently seen in MDS but their presence alone is not considered as presumptive of MDS because they can be seen in normal individuals:

- +8

- del(20q)

- -Y

42. C

Myelodysplastic syndrome with ring sideroblasts (MDS-RS), formally known as refractory anemia with ring sideroblasts (RARS), is a low grade MDS with an overall good prognosis.

Patients present with anemia and occasionally other cytopenias. The bone marrow shows dysplasia in the erythroid lineages with no dysplasia in the other lineages. Evaluation of the bone marrow aspirate with an iron stain shows the presence of ring sideroblasts accounting for at least 15% of erythroid precursors. Ring sideroblasts have 5 or more iron granules encircling one-third or more of the nucleus. Cases with multilineage dysplasia should be classified as myelodysplastic syndrome with ring sideroblasts with multilineage dysplasia (MDS-RS-MLD).

The presence of ring sideroblasts is closely associated with mutation of the spliceosome gene *SF3B1*. As such, the diagnosis of MDS-RS can be made with at least 5% ring sideroblasts in the presence of *SF3B1* or in the presence of 15% ring sideroblasts regardless of *SF3B1* mutation status.

The peripheral blood should contain less than 1% blasts and the bone marrow should contain less than 5% blasts. Cases with 1% blasts in the peripheral blood (measured on two separate occasions) should be classified as myelodysplastic syndrome unclassifiable (MDS-U). Cases with higher blast counts or Auer rods should be classified as myelodysplastic syndrome with excess blasts (MDS-EB).

43. C

The diagnosis of chronic myeloid leukemia (CML) is defined by the presence of the Philadelphia chromosome. The Philadelphia chromosome results from a reciprocal translocation of the long arms of chromosomes 9 and 22; t(9;22) 9q34;q11.2.

This translocation causes the *ABL1* gene, located on chromosome 9, to fuse with the *BCR* gene on chromosome 22 and results in the formation of the *BCR-ABL1* fusion gene which encodes the BCR-ABL1 oncoprotein. BCR-ABL1 has enhanced tyrosine kinase activity, which can be targeted by tyrosine kinase inhibitors such as imatinib.

BCR stands for breakpoint cluster region and *ABL1* is an oncogene known as Abelson murine leukemia viral oncogene. In the majority of CML cases, the breakpoint occurs in the major breakpoint cluster region (M-BCR), and results in the abnormal fusion protein p210.

A break in the minor breakpoint region (m-BCR) results in a shorter fusion protein, p190 and is most frequently seen in Philadelphia chromosome-positive B-lymphoblastic leukemia/lymphoma. These patients also benefit from the addition of tyrosine kinase inhibitors to their chemotherapy.

In rare cases of CML, the breakpoint region occurs in the μ-BCR region and results in a larger fusion protein, p230. These patients tend to have more prominent neutrophilic maturation or thrombocytosis.

Very rare cases of CML have the p190 protein and these cases show morphologic features similar to chronic myelomonocytic leukemia (CMML).

44. B

If untreated, chronic myeloid leukemia, *BCR-ABL1* positive, (CML), typically begins with a prolonged, indolent "chronic phase" (CP), followed by a more aggressive "accelerated phase" (AP). This phase may be fatal or may further progress into "blast phase" (BP) which is full progression to acute leukemia. Some patients may progress from CP immediately to BP. Progression through these phases is accompanied by certain clinical, morphologic and/or molecular genetic findings.

With the use of tyrosine kinase inhibitor (TKI) therapy, the majority of patients can remain in

CP for decades. Nevertheless, close monitoring of patients for progression is essential so that appropriate therapy may be initiated as soon as possible.

The accelerated phase of CML has the following features:

- Persistent or unresponsive white blood cell count (>10 x 10^9/L)
- Persistent or increasing splenomegaly, unresponsive to therapy
- Persistent thrombocytosis (>1000 x 10^9/L), unresponsive to therapy
- ≥ 20% basophils in the peripheral blood
- 10–19% blasts in the peripheral blood or bone marrow
- Additional clonal chromosomal abnormalities:
  - ○ Presence of a second Philadelphia chromosome
  - ○ +8
  - ○ i(17q)
  - ○ +19
  - ○ Complex karyotype (>3 abnormalities)
  - ○ Abnormalities of 3q26.2
  - ○ Any new clonal chromosomal abnormality that arises during therapy

Recently, additional provisional criteria for AP, based on response to TKI therapy, have been proposed:

- Failure to achieve complete hematologic remission with the first TKI
- Any resistance (failure to achieve hematologic, cytogenetic, or molecular resistance) to two sequential TKI's
- Occurrence of two or more point mutations in BCR-ABL1 during TKI therapy

The presence of ≥20% blasts in the peripheral blood or bone marrow, or the presence of an extramedullary proliferation of blasts is diagnostic of blast phase of CML. In addition, the detection of focal clusters or sheets of blasts that occupy a significant portion of the bone marrow (such as an entire intertrabecular region) are considered presumptive evidence of blast phase.

Blast phase of CML is most frequently of myeloid lineage, resembling acute myeloid leukemia (70–80%), but can be also be of lymphoblastic lineage, resembling acute lymphoblastic leukemia (20–30% of cases). Furthermore, blast phase of myeloid lineage can have monocytic, megakaryocytic and/or erythroid differentiation. Rare cases of development of acute promyelocytic leukemia in BP have also been reported.

45. C

The diagnosis of chronic myeloid leukemia, BCR-ABL1 positive, (CML), requires detection of BCR-ABL1 in the presence of certain clinicopathologic findings.

The disease is most commonly seen in older male patients (median age at diagnosis, 65 years). Clinically, patients may present with fatigue, weight loss, night sweats and early satiety related to splenomegaly and/or hepatomegaly. Lymphadenopathy is uncommon and, if present, should be biopsied to exclude the presence of blast phase of CML.

Of note, a significant number of patients (approximately 50%) with CML are completely asymptomatic and the disease is discovered incidentally during a work up for other reasons.

The peripheral blood and complete blood count shows leukocytosis composed predominantly of neutrophils with left shifted maturation (numerous immature forms). The predominant immature form is the myelocyte (resulting in a "myelocyte bulge" in the differential). Basophilia and eosinophilia are also common. Anemia is often present and platelets are either normal or mildly elevated.

Circulating blasts may be present but are usually less than 10% of white blood cells. The presence of 10–19% blasts is consistent with accelerated phase of CML and the presence of ≥ 20% blasts is consistent with blast phase of CML.

Rarely, the leukocytosis will be predominantly composed of segmented neutrophils, prompting consideration of chronic neutrophilic leukemia (CNL). These cases are associated with the p230 fusion protein. CNL is a rare myeloproliferative neoplasm that lacks BCR-ABL1 and is highly associated with the presence of an activating point mutation in the CSF3R gene. As such, any case of suspected CNL should undergo testing for BCR-ABL1 and evaluation of the CSF3R gene before diagnosis.

Absolute monocytosis (> 1 x 10^9/L) may be seen and may prompt consideration of chronic myelomonocytic leukemia (CMML), but in contrast to CMML, dysplasia is not present and the total percentage of monocytes is usually less than 10%. These cases are associated with the p190 fusion protein. As such, cases of suspected CMML should be investigated for the presence of BCR-ABL1 before diagnosis.

Rarely, leukocytosis will be minimal and thrombocytosis may be high enough to prompt consideration of essential thrombocythemia (ET). These cases are also associated with p230 fusion protein. As such, testing for BCR-ABL1 should be performed in any case of suspected ET.

The bone marrow is hypercellular (often approaching 100% cellularity) and is predominantly composed of neutrophils and myelocytes. A 5–10-cell layer of maturing myeloid cells may be seen around the bony trabeculae ("paratrabecular cuffing"). Basophilia and eosinophilia are often present. There is no dysplasia. Megakaryocytes may be normal in number or elevated and are often small with hypolobated nuclei (referred to as "dwarf megakaryocytes"). Histiocytes with expanded "sky-blue" cytoplasm, resembling Gaucher cells (referred to as Pseudo Gaucher cells) are frequently present. The presence of these cells is thought to be due to excess phospholipids and increased cellular turnover; however, it has been shown that these cells harbor BCR-ABL1 and are part of the malignant clone. Reticulin fibrosis may be present in 30–40% of cases.

46. A

Polycythemia vera (PV), primary myelofibrosis (PMF) and essential thrombocythemia (ET) are all associated with presence of JAK2 mutation. However, the JAK2 mutation is seen in essentially 100% of PV. It is seen in approximately half of patients with either PMF or ET.

The activating point mutation JAK2 V617F is seen in about 95% of cases of PV. The remaining cases are associated with a mutation in exon 12 of JAK2.

47. B

The detection of JAK2 V617F, mutated CALR and/or mutated MPL helps establish the diagnosis of a myeloproliferative neoplasm (MPN), but each is nonspecific. The clinical, laboratory and morphologic data of each case must be closely evaluated to properly classify the disease.

In polycythemia vera (PV), JAK2 V617F or a mutation in exon 12 of the JAK2 gene is found in essentially 100% of cases. Rarely, an additional mutation will also be found in the MPL gene. A homozygous mutation for JAK2 V617F is most often seen in PV, but is rarely seen in other MPN's (most often heterozygous).

In primary myelofibrosis (PMF) JAK2 V617F is found in approximately 50–60% of cases. A mutation in CALR is found in 25–30% of cases, and a mutation in MPL is found in 5–10% of cases.

The presence of a sole mutation in CALR is associated with a good prognosis in PMF, while the lack of any of the above mutations ("triple-negative" PMF) is associated with a poor prognosis.

In essential thrombocythemia (ET), JAK2 V617 is found in 50–60% of cases, mutated CALR is found in 25–30% and mutated MPL is found in 3–5%.

48. C

It has been recognized that two distinct phases of primary myelofibrosis (PMF) exist: an early pre-fibrotic phase and the classical fibrotic phase (also known as the overt fibrotic phase).

In the overt fibrotic phase of PMF, the peripheral blood shows leukoerythroblastosis with numerous dacrocytes (tear drop-shaped red blood cells) and large, abnormal platelets. Rarely circulating megakaryocyte nuclei may be observed.

Bone marrow cellularity varies with the stage of the disease. Hypercellularity is often seen in the early, pre-fibrotic phases and hypocellularity with near complete absence of hematopoiesis may be seen in the later stages of the fibrotic phases.

Nevertheless, all phases have increased megakaryocyte proliferation with atypical megakaryocyte morphology. The megakaryocytes often vary in size (a feature that helps in differentiation from essential thrombocythemia, where megakaryocytes are large and of uniform size). The cells vary from small to large with pleomorphic, bizarre nuclei containing "cloudlike" or "balloon-like "nuclear lobations. As the disease progresses, the megakaryocytes have a higher nuclear: cytoplasmic ratio and hyperchromatic nuclei. The megakaryocytes also show abnormal localization adjacent to the trabeculae and may show clustering. The remaining lineages are increased in the early phase and become decreased during progression to overt fibrotic stage.

A defining feature of overt fibrotic PMF is the presence of significant (grade 2–3) reticulin or collagen fibrosis which can be visualized with the use of reticulin and trichrome stains, respectively. Other morphologic signs of bone marrow fibrosis include the presence of dilated bone marrow sinuses, which may contain megakaryocytes and other immature hematopoietic cells (intrasinusoidal hematopoiesis). New bone formation and osteosclerosis (thickening of the bony trabeculae) may also be seen.

Dysplasia is not present and blasts are generally not increased. The presence of 10–19% blasts in the peripheral blood or bone marrow is consistent with accelerated phase of PMF, and the presence of ≥20% blasts is consistent with transformation to acute myeloid leukemia.

49. C
Mast cells can be visualized with the special stains Giemsa and chloroacetate. They are also positive for mast cell tryptase, chymase and CD117.

The presence of aberrant expression of CD2 and CD25 is indicative of a neoplastic mast cell population.

50. A
Atypical chronic myeloid leukemia, *BCR-ABL1* negative, (aCML)is a myelodysplastic/myeloproliferative neoplasm that contains left-shifted leukocytosis and resembles chronic myeloid leukemia. However, aCML is distinguished by the presence of marked dysplasia and the lack of *BCR-ABL1*. In addition, basophilia and monocytosis are not present.

51. C
B lymphoblastic leukemia/lymphoma with t(5;14)(q31;q32.3); *IL-3-IGH* is a rare neoplasm in which the *IL3* gene on chromosome 5 is juxtaposed with the *IGH* gene on chromosome 14. This results in constitutive overexpression of the *IL3* gene and results in marked peripheral blood eosinophilia. The degree of eosinophilia may be significant enough to obscure the lymphoblast population and cause toxic effects secondary to degranulation (cardiac effects, *etc.*).

52. B
B lymphoblastic leukemia/lymphoma with t(v;11q23);*KMT2A* (formally *MLL*) rearranged frequently occurs in infants. The partner gene is variable (v) but the most common translocation seen is t(4;11)(q21;q23). The result is aberrant regulation of the *KMT2A* (formally *MLL*) gene. These cases have a poor prognosis and tend to have high white blood cell counts and central nervous system involvement at diagnosis. The lymphoblasts are often CD10-negative and CD19-positive and show aberrant expression of the myeloid markers CD15 and CD65.

53. D
B lymphoblastic leukemia/lymphoma with t(12;21)(p13;q22); *ETV6-RUNX1* is the most common form of B lymphoblastic leukemia/lymphoma in children. It is not seen in infants and is extremely rare in adults. It is associated with a very favorable prognosis.

54. A
B lymphoblastic leukemia/lymphoma with t(9;22)(q34.1;q11.2); *BCR-ABL1* is more frequently seen in adult patients and it is the most frequently observed chromosomal abnormality in this patient population. It is associated with a poor prognosis. In the majority of cases, the *BCR-ABL1* fusion results in expression of the 190 kDa fusion protein, p190 (as opposed to the p210 protein most commonly seen in chronic myeloid leukemia). The prognosis of the disease is improved by the addition of tyrosine kinase inhibitor therapy to the therapeutic regimen.

55. C
Diagnosis of T lymphoblastic leukemia/lymphoma can be difficult due to the high propensity of the neoplastic T-lymphoblasts to aberrantly lose or gain T-cell antigen expression as well as the propensity other types of leukemia (such as acute myeloid leukemia) to aberrantly express T-cell antigens.

The diagnosis can be made by detection of antigens associated with immaturity in combination with detection of antigens associated with T-cell differentiation. The most commonly encountered antigens of immaturity are CD34, TdT, CD1a and HLA-DR (although this antigen is also seen in mature B-cells, monocytes and activated T-cells).

Cytoplasmic expression of CD3 (cCD3) is considered to be the most specific antigen for T-cell lineage.

56. D

Rare cases of T-cell lymphoblastic leukemia/lymphoma show a very primitive immunophenotype similar to early T-precursor cells in the thymus and/or bone marrow. These cases are referred to as early T-cell precursor lymphoblastic leukemia (ETP-ALL) and are associated with a poor prognosis.

These cases express TdT, CD34 and HLA-DR, and always express CD7, which is in fact one of the earliest markers expressed during T-cell differentiation. They also express cytoplasmic CD3 and show characteristic dim expression of CD5. They are often negative for CD1a and CD8. They characteristically express myeloid-associated antigens such as CD13, CD33 and CD117 (which may be associated with mutation of the *FLT3* gene). However, these cases should not be classified as mixed phenotype acute leukemia, because they do not express myeloperoxidase.

Mature B-Cell Lymphomas, Plasma Cell Neoplasms and Hodgkin Lymphoma: Questions 1–50

1. The following are true regarding follicular lymphoma:
   A. Follicular lymphoma is the most common lymphoma in the United States and Western Europe
   B. Typically has a fulminant onset
   C. Some cases progress to Hodgkin lymphoma
   D. Most patients have widespread disease at diagnosis

2. All of the following are histologic features of follicular lymphoma involving lymph nodes except:
   A. Effacement of lymph node architecture
   B. A well-demarcated mantle zone
   C. Absent or scanty tingible body macrophages
   D. Loss of polarity of the germinal center

3. The follicles in a case of follicular lymphoma are expected to be positive for
   A. CD10
   B. Bcl 6
   C. Bcl 2
   D. All of the above

4. Characteristic features of pediatric follicular lymphoma include
   A. High histologic grade
   B. Poor prognosis
   C. Widespread disseminated disease at diagnosis
   D. Frequent Bcl 2 positivity

5. Which of the following are features of primary cutaneous follicular center lymphoma (PCFCL)?
   A. PCFCL is the most common extranodal B-cell lymphoma
   B. Most often, the head and neck area are involved
   C. Dissemination to extracutaneous sites is very frequent
   D. Almost all cases are Bcl 2 positive

6. Follicular lymphoma is characterized by the following cytogenetic abnormality:
   A. t(8;14)
   B. t(14;18)
   C. t(15;17)
   D. t(11;14)

7. All of the following regarding chronic lymphocytic leukemia/small lymphocytic lymphoma (CLL/SLL) are true except:
   A. CLL/SLL is the most common leukemia in Western countries
   B. Radiation exposure does not increase the risk of developing CLL/SLL
   C. Most patients at presentation have fever and weight loss
   D. CLL/SLL patients are typically over 50 years of age

8. A characteristic feature of lymph node involved by CLL/SLL is:
   A. Effacement of lymph node architecture with presence of large and small cells
   B. Presence of pseudofollicles
   C. Marked increase in vascularity
   D. Large cells resembling Reed-Sternberg cells

9. The typical immunophenotype of CLL/SLL tumor cells includes:
   A. Bright expression of surface Ig and B-cell markers, along with positivity for CD5 and CD23
   B. Dim expression of surface Ig and B-cell markers, along with positivity for CD5 and CD23
   C. CD10, CD20 and CD5 positivity
   D. Cyclin D1, CD20 and CD5 positivity

10. Which of the following imparts a better prognosis for patients with CLL/SLL?
    A. CD38 negativity
    B. ZAP-70 positivity

C. Presence of Trisomy 12

D. Lymphocyte doubling time of 8 months

11. Mantle cell lymphoma is characterized by
    A. Low-grade behavior
    B. Marked female preponderance
    C. Localized disease at time of diagnosis
    D. Unlikely transformation to large cell lymphoma

12. Histologic features characteristic of mantle cell lymphoma include
    A. A heterogeneous population of lymphocytes
    B. A monotonous population of lymphocytes
    C. Marked increase in plasma cells
    D. Multinucleated giant cells

13. Mantle cell lymphoma should be positive for all of the following markers except:
    A. Cyclin D1
    B. CD 20
    C. CD 10
    D. CD 5

14. Which of the following is true for mantle cell lymphoma?
    A. The blastoid variant is a less aggressive form of mantle cell lymphoma
    B. Mantle cell lymphoma is positive for t(11;14)
    C. Proliferation centers are an expected finding in lymph nodes involved by mantle cell lymphoma
    D. Pleomorphic variant of mantle cell lymphoma imparts better prognosis

15. Which of the following is true for blastoid variant of mantle cell lymphoma?
    A. Most cases are cyclin D1 negative
    B. Majority of cases are Sox11 positive
    C. Most cases are CD5 negative
    D. Ki67 index is typically below 20%

16. Which of the following are seen in typical cases of marginal zone B-cell lymphoma?
    A. Minimal plasmacytic diffrentiation
    B. Minimal risk of transformation to diffuse large B-cell lymphoma (DLBCL)
    C. Aberrant expression of CD 43 in approximately 90% of cases
    D. Bone marrow involvement in 10–20% of cases

17. Which of the following is not a risk factor for the development of extranodal marginal zone lymphoma (MALT lymphoma)?
    A. Sjogren's syndrome
    B. Pernicious anemia
    C. Helicobacter pylori infection
    D. Hashimoto's thyroiditis

18. The cytogenetic abnormality often associated with MALT lymphoma is:
    A. t(14;18)
    B. t(11;18)
    C. t(15;17)
    D. t(8;14)

19. All of the following are features of splenic marginal zone lymphoma except:
    A. Lymphoma cells in the peripheral blood with circumferential villi
    B. Splenomegaly
    C. Involvement of splenic hilar lymph nodes by lymphoma
    D. Involvement of the bone marrow by lymphoma

20. The following are all features of nodal marginal zone lymphoma except:
    A. Tumor cells are CD79a positive
    B. Tumor cells are Bcl2 positive
    C. Tumor cells are CD10 positive
    D. Tumor cells are Bcl6 negative

21. Among the following epidemiological subtypes of Burkitt lymphoma, the one most often associated with EBV infection is
    A. Endemic type
    B. Sporadic type
    C. Immunodeficiency-associated type
    D. None of the above

22. All of the following are characteristic histologic features of Burkitt lymphoma except
    A. Diffuse growth pattern
    B. Starry sky appearance
    C. Large cells with inconspicuous nucleoli
    D. High mitotic rate

23. Which of the following positive immunohistochemical stains should make one reconsider a diagnosis of Burkitt lymphoma?
    A. CD10 positivity
    B. Bcl2 positivity

C. Bcl 6 positivity

D. CD20 positivity

24. Which of the following translocations may be seen in Burkitt lymphoma?

A. t(8;14)

B. t(2;8)

C. t(8;22)

D. All of the above

25. Which of the following is a true statement regarding lymphoplasmacytic lymphoma (LPL)?

A. It is synonymous with Waldenström macroglobulinemia

B. This is a high-grade lymphoma

C. It is associated with hepatitis C infection

D. It is not known to transform to a high-grade lymphoma

26. Which of the following regarding LPL is true?

A. This is an intermediate to high-grade lymphoma

B. It does not transform to diffuse large B-cell lymphoma

C. There are three main variants of LPL, lymphoplasmacytoid, lymphoplasmacytic and polymorphous

D. It is associated with bone marrow eosinophilia

27. Regarding diffuse large B-cell lymphoma (DLBCL) which of the following is false?

A. This is the most common lymphoma

B. This is a high-grade lymphoma

C. Bone marrow involvement at diagnosis is very common

D. Bone marrow if involved may demonstrate a lower grade of lymphoma

28. Which of the following typically does not transform to diffuse large B-cell lymphoma?

A. Mantle cell lymphoma

B. chronic lymphocytic leukemia

C. Follicular lymphoma

D. lymphoplasmacytic lymphoma

29. Which of the following immunophenotypic findings is consistent with a germinal center B-cell-like immunophenotype in diffuse large B-cell lymphoma (GCB DLBCL)?

A. CD10 (+)

B. CD10 (-), BCL6 (+), MUM-1 (+)

C. CD10 (-), BCL6 (-), MUM-1 (+)

D. CD10 (-), BCL6 (-), MUM-1 (-)

30. Diffuse large B-cell lymphoma may demonstrate positivity for all of the following immunostains except

A. CD3

B. ALK-1

C. CD30

D. CD5

31. Which of the following variants of diffuse large B-cell lymphoma (DLBCL) is not associated with EBV infection?

A. DLBCL associated with chronic inflammation

B. Intravascular large B-cell lymphoma

C. Primary effusion lymphoma

D. Lymphomatoid granulomatosis

32. Which of the following is not a typical feature of primary mediastinal large B-cell lymphoma?

A. Diffuse growth pattern of tumor cells with varying degrees of sclerosis

B. Cells with pale/clear cytoplasm

C. CD30 positivity in majority of cases

D. Surface light chain restriction

33. Which of the following is true regarding plasmablastic lymphoma?

A. This is a low-grade tumor

B. CD20 is strongly positive in most cases

C. Ki67 proliferation index is high (>70% in most cases)

D. CD138 is negative in most cases

34. Regarding primary diffuse large B-cell lymphoma of the CNS, which is true?

A. Lesions may spontaneously disappear

B. Most lesions affect the spinal cord

C. HIV positivity in affected patients is common

D. Pan B-cell markers such as CD20 are consistently negative

35. Primary effusion lymphoma patients may be infected with:

A. HIV

B. EBV

C. HHV-8

D. All of the above

36. All of the following are features of hairy cell leukemia except:
    A. The disease involves the red pulp of the spleen
    B. There is leukocytosis
    C. Monocytopenia occurs
    D. Bone marrow aspiration may result in a dry tap

37. All of the following markers are expected to be positive in hairy cell leukemia except:
    A. Annexin 1
    B. CD25
    C. CD103
    D. CD3

38. A distinct feature seen in hairy cell leukemia-variant but not in hairy cell leukemia is:
    A. Splenomegaly
    B. Circulating neoplastic lymphocytes in the peripheral blood
    C. Prominent nucleoli
    D. Similar response to treatment

39. All of the following are features of B-cell lymphoma, unclassifiable with features intermediate between diffuse large B-cell lymphoma and Burkitt lymphoma except:
    A. Aggressive clinical course
    B. Diffuse growth pattern with starry sky appearance
    C. High percentage of patients with disseminated disease
    D. Most patients will have normal cytogenetics

40. Thesaurocytes are:
    A. Plasma cells with flame shaped cytoplasm
    B. Plasma cells with ground glass cytoplasm
    C. Plasma cell with intra nuclear inclusion
    D. Binucleated plasma cells

41. Quantification of paraprotein in monoclonal gammopathy is done from:
    A. Serum protein electrophoresis
    B. Serum immunofixation
    C. Urine immunofixation
    D. Serum free light chain assay

42. Causes of a band in either the β or γ region on serum protein electrophoresis but negative serum immunofixation study include all of the following except:
    A. Bisalbuminemia
    B. Band due to fibrinogen
    C. Band due to hemoglobin-haptoglobin complex
    D. Band due to high levels of transferrin

43. A patient has a serum kappa to lambda light chain ratio of 3:1 (normal, 0.26–1.65). All other investigations (pathologic and radiologic) are negative for monoclonal gammopathy. A possible explanation for this isolated abnormality is:
    A. Nonsecretory myeloma
    B. Smoldering myeloma
    C. Renal failure
    D. Liver failure

44. Which of the following feature/s point(s) against a diagnosis of monoclonal gammopathy of undetermined significance (MGUS)?
    A. A 3% clonal population of plasma cells in the bone marrow
    B. Renal dysfunction due to polycystic kidney disease, diagnosed at birth
    C. Anemia
    D. A paraprotein level of 5g/L

45. Neoplastic plasma cells characteristically express which of the following?
    A. CD20
    B. CD19
    C. CD3
    D. CD56

46. In which of the following subtypes of Hodgkin lymphoma may nodules be seen under low-power microscopic examination?
    A. Lymphocyte rich classical Hodgkin lymphoma
    B. Nodular lymphocyte predominant Hodgkin lymphoma
    C. Nodular sclerosis classical Hodgkin lymphoma
    D. All of the above

47. Which of the following neoplastic cell types is not expected to be seen in a case of classical Hodgkin lymphoma?
    A. Reed-Sternberg cell
    B. L&H cell

C. Lacunar cell

D. Mummified cell

48. The immunophenotype most consistent with Reed-Sternberg cells in a case of Hodgkin lymphoma is:

A. Positivity for CD45, CD15 and CD30

B. Positivity for CD45, CD20 and Pax5

C. Negativity for CD45, weak positivity for Pax5 and positivity for CD15 and CD30 in a membrane and Golgi pattern

D. Negativity for CD45, CD15 and CD30

49. The immunophenotype most consistent with LP cells (popcorn cells) in nodular lymphocyte predominant Hodgkin lymphoma is:

A. Positivity for CD45, CD15 and CD30

B. Positivity for CD45 and negativity for CD15 and CD30

C. Positivity for CD15 and CD30 and negativity for CD20

D. Negativity for CD45, CD15 and CD30

50. Which of the following is not a subtype of classical Hodgkin lymphoma?

A. Nodular sclerosis

B. Eosinophil rich

C. Lymphocyte depleted

D. Lymphocyte rich

Answers to Chapter 5

1. D	14. B	27. C	40. B
2. B	15. B	28. A	41. A
3. D	16. D	29. A	42. A
4. A	17. B	30. A	43. C
5. B	18. B	31. B	44. C
6. B	19. A	32. D	45. D
7. C	20. C	33. C	46. D
8. B	21. A	34. A	47. B
9. B	22. C	35. D	48. C
10. A	23. B	36. B	49. B
11. D	24. D	37. D	50. B
12. B	25. C	38. C	
13. C	26. C	39. D	

Answers to Chapter 5 (with Explanations)

1. D

   Follicular lymphoma occurs due to neoplastic transformation of germinal center B-cells. It is the second most common non-Hodgkin lymphoma in the United States and Western Europe. It is seen less often in Asia and developing countries. The cervical and inguinal lymph nodes are most often affected. The disease typically is insidious in onset. Most patients have widespread disease at diagnosis. Follicular lymphoma typically has an indolent clinical course. Some cases (approx. 30%) progress to diffuse large B-cell lymphoma (DLBCL)

2. B

   Lymph nodes involved by follicular lymphoma demonstrate complete or partial loss of normal architecture. Neoplastic follicles are present which are typically closely packed and of uniform size. The mantle zone is faint or absent. The follicles have little mitotic activity as well as reduced or absent tingible body macrophages. Centrocytes and centroblasts are randomly distributed. Thus there is loss of polarity. The architectural pattern of the disease is subdivided into follicular (>75% follicular), follicular and diffuse (25–75% follicular) minimally follicular (<25% follicular) and diffuse (a diffuse area is an area of tissue completely lacking follicles defined by lack of CD21/CD23 staining for follicular dendritic cells). Follicular lymphoma is graded from 1 to 3. In grade 1, there are 0–5 centroblasts/hpf, and in grade 3 there are >15 centroblasts/hpf. Grade 3 can be subdivided to 3a and 3b. In 3a some centrocytes are present. In 3b there are no centrocytes. Solid sheets of centroblasts occupy the affected area.

3. D

   The neoplastic follicles in follicular lymphoma stain positively for B-cell markers such as CD20 and markers associated with germinal center cells, such as CD10 and Bcl 6. Neoplastic follicles in follicular lymphoma should also stain for Bcl2.

   Reactive follicles are negative for Bcl2. Low-grade follicular lymphomas will typically have a low proliferation index (i.e. Ki67 <20%).

   High-grade follicular lymphomas (grade 3) can be CD10 negative, Bcl2 negative and have a higher proliferation index (Ki67>40%)

4. A

   Pediatric follicular lymphomas are typically a localized disease affecting neck nodes. The histologic grade is usually high. They are usually Bcl 2 negative. The usual translocation, t(14;18), is lacking. Prognosis is, however, good without disease progression.

5. B

   PCFCL is the second most common extranodal B-cell lymphoma after GI lymphomas. The head and neck area is most often involved. Although the skin lesions will increase in size if untreated, dissemination to extracutaneous sites is uncommon (10% or less). PCFCL may be Bcl2 negative.

6. B

   The majority of patients with follicular lymphoma exhibit the translocation t(14;18) (q32;q21). As a result of this translocation the Bcl2 gene is juxtaposed to the immunoglobulin heavy chain gene. This results in overproduction of Bcl2 protein. This blocks apoptosis.

7. C

   Chronic lymphocytic leukemia/small lymphocytic lymphoma (CLL/SLL) is the most common leukemia in the Western world. It also has the highest genetic predisposition. Most patients are asymptomatic at presentation. Some may present with features of autoimmune hemolytic anemia. Herpes zoster in an elderly patient may be a clue at times for an underlying CLL. Most patients are over 50 years of age at presentation. The absolute lymphocyte count is greater than 5000/mm3 of blood for at least 3 months.

8. B

When a lymph node is involved by CLL/SLL, then there is usually effacement of normal architecture with presence of mainly small cells. Pseudofollicles, which resemble vague nodules, are a characteristic finding. Pseudofollicles have proliferation centers that contain prolymphocytes (medium-sized cells with dispersed chromatin and small nucleoli) and paraimmunoblasts (large cells with dispersed chromatin and central nucleoli). Plasmacytoid differentiation may be observed.

9. B

In CLL/SLL the tumor cells are positive for B-cell markers (e.g. CD20, CD19). Surface immunoglobulin will demonstrate light chain restriction. Surface immunoglobulin and B-cell markers are typically dimly expressed. The tumors are also positive for CD5 and CD23. Mantle cell lymphoma typically is CD5 positive and CD23 negative. Please note, some cases of CLL may be positive for CD23 in a weak or partial manner.

10. A

CD38 positivity and ZAP-70 positivity are both considered to be poor prognostic markers for CLL/SLL. Individuals who have CLL/SLL and possess del 13q14 usually have a long survival time. It is the most frequent chromosomal abnormality seen in patients with CLL/SLL. Trisomy 12, deletion of 17p, and deletion of 11q are associated with a poor prognosis. Doubling of the absolute lymphocyte count in less than one year also implies poor prognosis.

CLL/SLL may undergo transformation to diffuse large B-cell lymphoma (3.5% of cases) or classical Hodgkin lymphoma (0.5% of cases). This high-grade transformation is referred to as "Richter's transformation."

11. D

Mantle cell lymphoma is an aggressive lymphoma. The median age of patients is 60 years with a male preponderance. Most patients at time of diagnosis are either stage III or IV (Ann Arbor staging). Mantle cell lymphoma typically does not transform to large cell lymphoma. Aggressive chemotherapy +/– stem cell transplantation is the preferred mode of treatment.

12. B

Mantle cell lymphoma is characterized by effacement of lymph node architecture by a monotonous population of cells. The proliferating cells

are small to medium lymphoid cells that resemble centrocytes. There is an increase in hyalinized blood vessels. The growth pattern may be nodular or diffuse or mantle zone pattern.

13. C

Mantle cell lymphoma is a B-cell tumor. Therefore, B-cell markers such as CD20, CD19 and Pax 5 should be positive. The tumors cells aberrantly express CD5 but not CD23. Surface immunoglobulins demonstrate light chain restriction. Cyclin D1 overexpression is a constant feature of mantle cell lymphoma. Mantle cell lymphoma is Bcl2 positive. It is negative for CD10 and Bcl 6.

14. B

Mantle cell lymphoma is characterized by t(11;14). There are several variants of mantle cell lymphoma. These include blastoid, pleomorphic, small cell, and marginal zone like. The blastoid and pleomorphic variants are considered to be aggressive variants. Proliferation centers are a feature of SLL not mantle cell lymphoma.

15. B

Blastoid variant of mantle cell lymphoma is an aggressive form of mantle cell lymphoma. Cyclin D1 is virtually always positive. Sox 11 is positive in majority of cases. Typically they are CD5 positive and CD23 negative. Some cases may be CD5 negative. As it is an aggressive lymphoma, Ki67 index should be high (i.e. well above 40%).

16. D

Marginal zone lymphoma exhibits a heterogeneous population of cells that include centrocyte-like cells, small lymphocytes, centroblasts, immunoblasts, and monocytoid B-cells (cells with abundant clear cytoplasm). Plasmacytic differentiation is common. The presence of monocytoid cells give the tumor a pink appearance. There is increased risk of transformation to diffuse large B-cell lymphoma. The gastrointestinal tract is the most common site of involvement, with the stomach representing the most common site of involvement. Bone marrow involvement is seen in 10–20% of cases. CD43 is seen in about 50% of cases. CD5, CD10 and cyclin D1 are all negative. There is no specific marker for marginal zone lymphoma.

17. B

Pernicious anemia predisposes to gastric carcinoma. H Pylori infection is associated with gastric extranodal marginal zone lymphoma (MALT lymphoma). Sjogren's syndrome is associated with salivary gland MALT lymphoma. Hashimoto's thyroiditis is associated with MALT lymphoma of the thyroid gland.

18. B

The translocation that is associated with extranodal marginal zone lymphoma (MALT lymphoma) is t(11;18). This translocation is most often seen in gastric MALT lymphomas (30–50% of cases). The incidence is much less in MALT lymphomas of other sites.

19. A

Splenic marginal zone lymphoma is a rare tumor. The tumor cells surround the white pulp of the spleen with effacement of the mantle zone. The tumor cells expand into the marginal zone. Splenic hilar lymph nodes and the bone marrow are often involved. Tumor cells may be seen in the peripheral blood with polar villi. Circumferential villi are a feature of hairy cell leukemia.

20. C

Nodal marginal zone lymphoma is a B-cell tumor. Therefore B-cell markers such as CD20, CD79a are expected to be positive. The tumor cells are typically Bcl2 positive and Bcl6 negative. CD5, CD10 and cyclin D1 are negative. CD43 may be aberrantly expressed.

21. A

Endemic type of Burkitt lymphoma is mostly seen in Africa and in children. Most often jaws and abdomen are involved. EBV is detected in most of these cases. The sporadic type is seen in both children and young adults. EBV infection is seen in about a third of cases. In immunodeficiency-associated Burkitt lymphoma EBV infection is seen in approximately 25% of cases.

22. C

Burkitt lymphoma is a high-grade tumor that typically has a diffuse growth pattern. Low-power examination reveals a starry sky appearance. The cells are medium-sized cells with prominent nucleoli.

23. B

Burkitt lymphoma is a B-cell tumor. Therefore, B-cell markers (e.g. CD20, CD79a) should be positive. Being of germinal center cell origin, Burkitt lymphoma is also positive for CD10 and BCL-6. BCL-2 is characteristically negative and its presence should prompt consideration of an alternative diagnosis. Ki-67 is extremely high, approaching 100%. TDT expression should also be evaluated to exclude B-lymphoblastic lymphoma, which may show morphologic and immunophenotypic similarities to Burkitt lymphoma.

24. D

Burkitt lymphoma patients may have any of the three translocations listed: t(8;14), t(2;8) and t(8;22). In t(8;14), the c-MYC gene on chromosome 8 and the Immunoglobulin Heavy Chain gene on chromosome 14 are rearranged. In t(2;8) the kappa gene on chromosome 2 is rearranged. In t(8;22) the lambda gene on chromosome 22 is rearranged.

25. C

Lymphoplasmacytic lymphoma (LPL) is a low-grade lymphoma with a familial predisposition (20%) and is also associated with hepatitis C infection. Serum monoclonal protein with hyperviscosity or cryoglobulinemia may be present. If the monoclonal protein is IgM and if the IgM concentration in serum is greater than 3g/l, then this is referred to as Waldenström macroglobulinemia.

26. C

Lymphoplasmacytic lymphoma (LPL) is a low-grade lymphoma and can transform to diffuse large B-cell lymphoma. There is involvement of the bone marrow and sometimes the lymph nodes and spleen. The morphology of LPL is characterized by the presence of a spectrum of cells. Small B lymphocytes, plasma cells, and plasmacytoid cells are seen. There may be an increase in histiocytes and mast cells.

There are three main histologic variants of LPL. These are lymphoplasmacytoid (here small lymphocytes predominate with presence of occasional plasma cells), lymphoplasmacytic (here small lymphocytes, plasmacytoid cells and plasma cells are all present) and polymorphous (here in addition there are some large cells).

27. C

Diffuse large B-cell lymphoma is the most common lymphoma. It accounts for about 30–40% of all non-Hodgkin lymphoma in adults. This is a high-grade lymphoma. Bone marrow involvement at diagnosis is low at approximately 10% of cases. Bone marrow if involved may demonstrate a lower grade of lymphoma. This phenomenon is referred to as discordant lymphoma.

28. A

Chronic lymphocytic leukemia/small lympho-cytic lymphoma, follicular lymphoma, marginal zone lymphoma, nodular lymphocyte predomi-nant Hodgkin lymphoma and lymphoplasma-cytic lymphoma can all transform to diffuse large B-cell lymphoma. Mantle cell lymphoma does not transform to DLBCL.

29. A

Diffuse large B-cell lymphoma (DLBCL) can be divided into two "cell of origin" (COO) sub-types based on gene expression profiling (GEP). The two subtypes are the Germinal Center B-cell (GCB) and Activated B-cell (ABC) subtypes. The GCB subtype is associated with better over-all survival. The ABC subtype may benefit from medications that target the NF-κB pathway and/or Bruton tyrosine kinase (BTK).

Many immunohistochemistry-based algorithms have been developed to approximate the cell of ori-gin in DLBCL. By immunohistochemistry, DLBCL may be divided into a "germinal center B-cell like (GCB)" or a "non-germinal center B-cell like (non-GCB)" subgroup. Various immunohistochemical algorithms have been developed for this purpose but the most commonly used is the "Han's algo-rithm". Using this algorithm, the following immu-nophenotypes are considered GCB-like:

A. CD10(+)
B. CD10(-), BCL-6(+), MUM-1 (-)

Cases which are CD10(-), BCL-6(+), MUM-1 (+) are considered to be non-GCB-like.
Expression of the marker in ≥30% neoplastic cells is considered "positive".
It is important to note that these subdivisions do not completely correlate (75% to 90% correlation) with the GCB and ABC subtypes defined by GEP. In addition, cases of DLBCL which co-express BCL2 and MYC by *immunohistochemistry* have recently been referred to as "Dual Expresser" type. These cases have a slightly worse prognosis than DLBCL without this immunophenotype, but a better prog-nosis than cases with rearrangements of MYC, BCL2, and/or BCL6 (double or triple hit lymphomas).

30. A

DLBCL is a B-cell tumor. Therefore B-cell mark-ers such as CD20, CD79a and Pax5 should be pos-itive. T-cell markers should be negative. However,

there exists entities, CD5 positive DLBCL and ALK positive DLBCL. CD30 is found to be pos-itive in about 30% of cases of DLBCL. CD10 positivity implies transformation from follicular lymphoma. Bcl2 is found to be positive in about 30% of cases and Bcl6 is positive more frequently.

31. B

Diffuse large B-cell lymphoma associated with chronic inflammation, lymphomatoid granulo-matosis, EBV positive diffuse large B-cell lym-phoma of the elderly, plasmablastic lymphoma and primary effusion lymphoma are associated with EBV infection.

32. D

Primary mediastinal large B-cell lymphoma is presumed to be of thymic B-cell origin. The dis-ease presents as an enlarging mass in the medias-tinum. Histology reveals a diffuse growth pattern with cells with pale or clear cytoplasm. There is usually some degree of sclerosis. The tumor is positive for B-cell markers. CD30 positivity is seen in about 80% of cases. The tumor cells lack surface immunoglobulin.

33. C

Plasmablastic lymphoma is a high-grade tumor. It is a variant of diffuse large B-cell lymphoma, occurring most commonly in HIV-positive patients. The tumor cells are typically negative for common B-cell markers such as CD20 and Pax5. CD79a may be positive but with weak intensity. Plasma cell associated markers such as CD38 and CD138 are strongly positive.

34. A

Primary diffuse large B-cell lymphoma of the CNS is not associated with a specific viral infec-tion. Most of the tumors are supratentorial in location, the most common site being the cere-brum. The tumor cells are positive for pan B-cell markers such as CD20. MUM1 is positive in the majority of cases (90%). CD10, Bcl2, and Bcl6 may be positive in varying degrees. The prolifer-ation index is usually high (>40%). These tumors are known to disappear spontaneously or with the administration of corticosteroids. This phenome-non is referred to as vanishing tumors.

35. D

Patients with primary effusion lymphoma are typically HIV-positive individuals who are also coinfected with HHV-8 and EBV. This lymphoma involves the body cavities. The cells are large with plasmablastic differentiation. This is a high-grade tumor.

36. B

Hairy cell leukemia is an indolent lymphoma of the bone marrow and spleen. In the spleen it affects the red pulp (forming "blood lakes"). In the peripheral blood, atypical lymphocytes with hairy cytoplasmic projections are seen. The patient typically has pancytopenia and monocytopenia. Attempts at bone marrow aspiration typically results in a dry tap. The bone marrow findings (mostly biopsy specimen) include increased reticulin and cells with pale clear cytoplasm (fried egg appearance).

37. D

Hairy cell leukemia (HCL) is a B-cell tumor. CD3, a T-cell marker is not expected to be positive. HCL is typically positive for CD11c, CD25, CD103, CD123 and Annexin 1.

38. C

Hairy cell leukemia-variant (HCL-V) has many similarities with HCL. HCL-V typically does not present with pancytopenia. In contrast, the white cell count is typically elevated. HCL-V patients may have anemia or thrombocytopenia but monocytopenia is not a characteristic feature. The tumor cells in HCL-V exhibit prominent nucleoli. The conventional chemotherapy used in HCL, if applied to HCL-V, yields poorer results.

39. D

B-cell lymphoma with features intermediate between diffuse large B-cell lymphoma and Burkitt lymphoma is an aggressive lymphoma. Majority of patients have disseminated disease at presentation. A subset of patients have rearrangement of the MYC gene in combination with rearrangement of the BCL2 or BCL6 gene ("double hit" lymphoma); rare patients have rearrangements of all three genes ("triple hit" lymphoma). Complex karyotype (>3 chromosomal abnormalities) is quite common.

Histology usually reveals diffuse growth pattern with starry sky appearance. Mitotic rate is high. Intermediate-sized cells with a spectrum of intermediate to large cells are seen.

In the updated 2016 World Health Classification, this disease category has been eliminated. Such cases are now referred to as "high-grade B-cell lymphoma, not otherwise specified (NOS)". All cases should be evaluated for MYC, BCL2, and BCL6 rearrangements. If present, the rearrangement should be listed in the diagnosis (e.g. "high grade B-cell lymphoma with MYC and BCL2 rearrangement").

40. B

Thesaurocytes are plasma cells with ground glass cytoplasm. It is very hard to distinguish reactive or normal plasma cells from neoplastic plasma cells from morphology alone. Trinucleated plasma cells and plasmablasts are certainly a feature of neoplastic plasma cells.

Intranuclear inclusions are referred to as Dutcher bodies. Immunoglobulin inclusions may be seen in the cytoplasm. When they appear as a grapelike cluster the cell is referred to as Mott cells. Flame shaped cytoplasm of plasma cells may denote IgA monoclonal gammopathy. None of these features is diagnostic for neoplastic plasma cells.

41. A

Quantification of paraprotein in a patient with monoclonal gammopathy is done from the serum protein electrophoresis study. It cannot be done from serum or urine immunofixation study.

42. A

Monoclonal proteins (or paraproteins) are typically seen in the γ region of serum protein electrophoresis, sometimes in the β region and rarely in the α-2 region. They do not migrate in the α-1 or albumin region.

Bisalbuminemia is considered when there are two albumin bands. This is a familial condition with no clinical significance.

If protein electrophoresis is performed on a plasma sample instead of a serum sample, fibrinogen produces a band between the β and γ region. If thrombin is added to the sample and the test is repeated the band disappears. Serum immunofixation will be negative.

Intravascular hemolysis results in the release of free hemoglobin which binds to haptoglobin. The hemoglobin-haptoglobin complex may produce a band in the α-2 area. Again serum immunofixation study is negative.

Patients with iron deficiency anemia will have high levels of transferrin. The abnormally high transferrin may result in a band seen in the β region.

Individuals with nephrotic syndrome have low total protein and low levels of albumin. The α-2 fraction as well as β globulin levels are high. These may result in bands. Naturally, serum immuno-fixation study is negative.

43. C

Quantitative serum assays for kappa and lambda free light chain are a very useful tool for diagnosing monoclonal gammopathy, especially light chain diseases. The rapid clearance of light chains by the kidney is significantly reduced in renal failure. The kappa to lambda ratio may be as high as 3:1. Therefore, patients with renal failure may have abnormally raised kappa to lambda ratio. If a patient has lambda light chain monoclonal gammopathy with renal failure then the relative increase in the kappa light chain will mask the abnormal kappa to lambda light chain ratio.

44. C

Monoclonal gammopathy of undetermined significance (MGUS) has a risk of progression to myeloma and the risk is about 1% per year. IgM MGUS may progress to lymphoplasmacytic lymphoma or Waldenström macroglobulinemia.

Features of MGUS include a paraprotein concentration less than 30g/L, a plasma cell population of less than 10% in the bone marrow and absence of end organ damage (manifesting as hypercalcemia, lytic bone lesions, anemia, and renal dysfunction). Renal dysfunction due to polycystic disease of the kidney cannot be attributed to MGUS or myeloma.

45. D

Plasma cells, both normal and neoplastic ones, express CD38 and CD138. Both normal and abnormal plasma cells are negative for CD20. Abnormal plasma cells are negative for CD19. In contrast, normal plasma cells are positive for CD19. Abnormal plasma cells may also be CD56 positive. Abnormal plasma cells should demonstrate cytoplasmic light chain restriction.

46. D

Nodules may be seen under low-power microscopic examination in all of the following

A. Lymphocyte rich classical Hodgkin lymphoma

B. Nodular lymphocyte predominant Hodgkin lymphoma

C. Nodular sclerosis classical Hodgkin lymphoma

47. B

Various neoplastic cells may be seen in classical Hodgkin lymphoma. These are Reed-Sternberg cells, mononuclear Hodgkin cells, lacunar cells, and mummified cells.

The Reed-Sternberg cell is a large cell with abundant cytoplasm and two mirror image nuclei. Each nuclei has an eosinophilic nucleolus. The mononuclear Hodgkin cell has similar features to that of a Reed-Sternberg cell but has only one nucleus. The lacunar cell has a cytoplasm that is retracted around the nucleus creating an empty space. The nucleus is single and hyperlobulated.

The mummified cell has a compact nucleus without any nucleoli. The cytoplasm is basophilic.

The L&H (lymphohistiocytic) cell, aka "popcorn" cell, is seen in nodular lymphocyte predominant Hodgkin lymphoma. These are large cells with hyperlobulated nuclei.

48. C

Reed-Sternberg cells in Hodgkin lymphoma are negative for CD45 and positive for CD15 and CD30. CD15 and CD30 stain the membrane and Golgi areas. Reed-Sternberg cells are positive for CD20 in 30–40% of cases. Pax5 stains Reed-Sternberg cells, weakly.

49. B

The L&H cells in NLPHL are CD20 positive, CD45 positive and negative for CD15 and CD30. CD20 highlights the nodules. The expanded meshwork of follicular dendritic cells is highlighted by CD21 and CD23. The L&H cells may be positive for EMA in about 50% of cases.

50. B

Hodgkin lymphoma is broadly categorized into nodular lymphocyte predominant Hodgkin lymphoma (NLPHL) and classical Hodgkin lymphoma (CHL). CHL is again subcategorized into nodular sclerosis, mixed cellularity, lymphocyte depleted and lymphocyte rich subtypes.

Mature T-Cell and NK-Cell Neoplasms: Questions 1–64

1. A 55-year-old Caucasian woman presents for evaluation of fatigue. The patient states that her symptoms have been present for approximately eight months and reports two episodes of cellulitis over the last year. Physical examination reveals mild splenomegaly; no skin lesions, lymphadenopathy, or other abnormalities are identified. Review of a complete blood count (CBC) and peripheral blood smear shows absolute neutropenia, normocytic, normochromic anemia, and mild absolute lymphocytosis composed of numerous large lymphocytes with abundant cytoplasm and prominent red-pink granules. Which of the following is the most likely diagnosis?
   A. T-cell prolymphocytic leukemia
   B. T-cell large granular lymphocytic leukemia
   C. Adult T-cell leukemia/lymphoma
   D. Aggressive NK-cell leukemia

2. The aforementioned patient undergoes bone marrow evaluation; immunohistochemical studies show an interstitial and intrasinusoidal infiltrate composed of CD4-, CD8+ cells. Flow cytometry performed on the specimen shows that the cells have the following immunophenotype:

   CD2+, CD3-, CD4-, CD5+, CD7-, CD8+, CD16+, CD56+, CD57-, CD94+.

   Which of the following is the most likely diagnosis?
   A. T-cell prolymphocytic leukemia
   B. T-cell large granular lymphocytic leukemia
   C. Chronic lymphoproliferative disorders of NK-cells
   D. Aggressive NK-cell leukemia

3. A 54-year-old man presents with a 6-month history of neutropenia. Review of a complete blood count and peripheral blood film shows absolute lymphocytosis composed predominantly of large granular lymphocytes (LGLs). Which of the following would most reliably distinguish the LGLs as natural killer (NK) cells?
   A. Expression of surface CD3 by flow cytometry
   B. Presence of a monoclonal rearrangement of the TCR-γ and TCR-β genes by PCR
   C. Expression of TCR αβ by flow cytometry
   D. Presence of a germline configuration of the TCR-γ and TCR-β genes by PCR

4. Which of the following is not a common characteristic of NK-cells?
   A. Cell surface expression of CD2
   B. Cell surface expression of CD3
   C. Cell surface expression of CD94
   D. Cell surface expression of neural cell adhesion molecule (N-CAM)

5. Which of the following findings would not be expected in a patient with T-cell large granular lymphocytic leukemia?
   A. Detection of Gram positive cocci on Gram stain of peripheral blood
   B. Detection of Rheumatoid factor (RF) by serology
   C. Detection of diffuse retroperitoneal lymphadenopathy on CT-scan
   D. Detection of thrombocytopenia on complete blood count

6. Which of the following would not be expected in the past medical history of a patient with T-cell large granular lymphocytic leukemia?
   A. History of HTLV-1 infection in childhood
   B. History of chronic lymphocytic leukemia
   C. History of bone marrow transplant
   D. History of Felty's syndrome

7. A 65-year-old Canadian man is admitted to the ICU with fever, weakness and a history of a 20-lb weight loss over the last 2 months. Physical examination and imaging studies show the presence of numerous maculopapular rashes, bilateral pleural effusions, diffuse lymphadenopathy and marked splenomegaly. A complete blood count and peripheral blood smear review shows the presence of marked leukocytosis (150 x10⁹/L) predominantly composed of atypical lymphocytes. Serologic studies for HIV, Hepatitis B and C and HTLV-1 are negative. The patient has no previous history of malignancy. Of the conditions listed here, which is the most likely diagnosis?
   A. T-cell large granular lymphocytic leukemia (T-LGLL)
   B. T-cell prolymphocytic leukemia (T-PLL)
   C. Sézary syndrome
   D. Adult T-cell leukemia/lymphoma (ATLL)

8. Which of the following is most likely to be seen in the peripheral blood smear of a patient with T-cell prolymphocytic leukemia?
   A. Medium-sized atypical lymphocytes with round to irregular nuclei, condensed chromatin, a prominent nucleolus and basophilic cytoplasm containing numerous cytoplasmic "blebs"
   B. Medium-sized atypical lymphocytes with round nuclei, condensed chromatin and abundant cytoplasm containing numerous large, azurophilic granules
   C. Medium-sized atypical lymphocytes with irregular polylobated "flower-like" nuclei, hypercondensed chromatin and basophilic cytoplasm with occasional vacuoles
   D. Medium-sized atypical lymphocytes with irregular "cerebriform" nuclei, dispersed chromatin and minimal cytoplasm

9. Which of the following would most likely be seen in the bone marrow of a patient with T-cell prolymphocytic leukemia?
   A. Sinusoidal lymphocytic infiltrate; positive for TIA-1
   B. Interstitial lymphocytic infiltrate; positive for CD94
   C. Diffuse lymphocytic infiltrate; positive for CD30
   D. Diffuse lymphocytic infiltrate; positive for TCL-1

10. Which of the following flow cytometry findings would be expected in a patient with T-cell prolymphocytic leukemia?
    A. Dim expression of CD34
    B. Co-expression of CD8 and CD56
    C. Co-expression of CD4 and CD8
    D. Expression of CD1a

11. Which of the following genetic abnormalities would not be expected in a patient with T-cell prolymphocytic leukemia?
    A. Inversion of chromosome 14
    B. Trisomy of chromosome 8
    C. Loss of 11q23
    D. Isochrome 7q

12. Which of the following findings would not be an expected finding in a patient with adult T-cell leukemia/lymphoma (ATLL)?
    A. History of HTLV-1 infection
    B. History of recent kidney transplant
    C. History of recent *Pneumocystis jiroveci* pneumonia
    D. History of intravenous drug abuse

13. Which of the following would be an expected finding in a patient with adult T-cell leukemia/ lymphoma (ATLL)?
    A. Peripheral blood basophilia
    B. Hypocalcemia
    C. Lytic bone lesions
    D. Decreased LDH

14. Which of the following is the most common site of extranodal involvement in adult T-cell leukemia/lymphoma (ATLL)?
    A. Heart
    B. Liver
    C. Central nervous system
    D. Skin

15. A 65-year-old man presents with a rash on the bilateral arms and legs. No other symptoms are present. Physical examination and imaging studies show no lymphadenopathy, splenomegaly or other sites of disease. The peripheral blood and bone marrow show no abnormalities. A biopsy of one of the skin lesions shows a prominent dermal and periadnexal infiltrate composed of small to intermediate-sized lymphocytes with irregular,

occasional cerebriform nuclei and condensed chromatin. No epidermotropism is identified. Immunohistochemical studies show the lymphocytes to be positive for CD2, CD3, CD4, CD5 and CD25; they are negative for CD7, CD8, CD26, CD56, CD57 and TCL1. Serology for HTLV-1 is positive. Which of the following is the most accurate statement?

A. The patient has mycosis fungoides.

B. This patient has adult T-cell leukemia/lymphoma, smoldering variant.

C. The patient has cutaneous T-cell prolymphocytic leukemia.

D. The patient has adult T-cell leukemia/lymphoma, lymphomatous variant.

16. A cutaneous biopsy from a 56-year-old man with multiple papules and ulcerating nodules shows the presence of a dermal infiltrate composed of small to intermediate-sized atypical lymphocytes with irregular nuclei. Focal epidermotropism is present. Which of the following findings would be most consistent with a cutaneous adult T-cell leukemia/lymphoma?

A. Detection of CD3 and TIA-1

B. Detection of CD3 and CD25

C. Detection of CD4 and CD8

D. Detection of CD3 and TCL-1

17. Which of the following morphologic findings would not be an expected finding in an excisional lymph node biopsy from a patient with adult T-cell leukemia/lymphoma?

A. Diffuse proliferation of medium to large-sized atypical lymphocytes with highly irregular nuclei admixed with giant cells showing bizarre nuclear contours

B. Paracortical expansion by small to medium-sized atypical lymphocytes admixed with numerous Hodgkin/Reed-Sternberg-like cells

C. Diffuse proliferation of medium to large-sized atypical lymphocytes with irregular nuclei and abundant, clear cytoplasm admixed with numerous eosinophils and plasma cells with proliferation of high endothelial venules in the background

D. Intrasinusoidal and subcapsular infiltrate of large atypical lymphocytes with abundant cytoplasm, anaplastic, kidney/

horseshoe-shape nuclei and prominent nucleoli

18. Which of the following molecular genetic findings would be most useful in establishing a diagnosis of adult T-cell leukemia/lymphoma?

A. Detection of a monoclonal rearrangement of the *TCR-γ* and *TCR-β* genes by PCR

B. Detection of a complex karyotype

C. Detection of germline configuration of the *TCR-γ* and *TCR-β* genes by PCR

D. Detection of HTLV-1 provirus DNA in clonal cells

19. Which of the following locations is least likely to be involved in a patient with the acute variant of adult T-cell leukemia/lymphoma?

A. Skin

B. Bone marrow

C. Peripheral blood

D. Lymph nodes

20. A 19-year-old man presents with a 3-month history of weight loss, fever and night sweats. He has a past medical history of renal transplant as a child, but no history of prior malignancy. Physical examination and imaging studies show marked splenomegaly, but no lymphadenopathy, skin rashes or other areas of disease. The peripheral blood shows thrombocytopenia but no other abnormalities. Flow cytometry on the peripheral blood shows no atypical cell populations. Of the choices listed below, which is the most likely diagnosis?

A. T-cell large granular lymphocytic leukemia

B. T-cell prolymphocytic leukemia

C. Adult T-cell leukemia/lymphoma

D. Hepatosplenic T-cell lymphoma

21. What would be the most expected finding in the bone marrow of a patient with hepatosplenic T-cell lymphoma?

A. Diffuse infiltrate, positive for CD3 and TCL-1

B. Intrasinusoidal infiltrate, positive for CD3 and TIA-1

C. Patchy infiltrate, positive for CD3 and CD25

D. Intrasinusoidal infiltrate, negative for CD3 and positive for TIA-1

22. Which of the following cytogenetic abnormalities would not be expected in a patient with hepatosplenic T-cell lymphoma?
    A. Deletion of chromosome 7q
    B. Multiple copies of isochrome 7q
    C. Deletion of chromosome Y
    D. Ring chromosome 7

23. Which of the following findings is most likely to be encountered in a patient with enteropathy-associated T-cell lymphoma (formally Type I enteropathy associated T-cell lymphoma)?
    A. Severe immune deficiency
    B. Recent solid organ transplant
    C. Concurrent gastric cancer
    D. Concurrent history of celiac disease

24. Which of the following macroscopic and microscopic findings would not be expected in a patient with enteropathy-associated T-cell lymphoma?
    A. Transmural infiltrate composed of medium to large atypical lymphocytes with irregular to anaplastic nuclei, dispersed chromatin and prominent nucleoli in a background of inflammation and necrosis
    B. Jejunal involvement by multiple small, ulcerating nodules
    C. Transmural infiltrate composed of medium-sized lymphocytes with round nuclei, condensed chromatin and a thin rim of pale cytoplasm
    D. Jejunal involvement by a large exophytic mass with extensive ulceration

25. Enteropathy associated T-cell lymphoma and monomorphic epitheliotropic intestinal T-cell lymphoma differ in all of the following except:
    A. Site of disease localization
    B. Morphology of neoplastic infiltrate
    C. Immunophenotype of neoplastic infiltrate
    D. Concomitant presence of celiac disease

26. Which of the following morphologic and immunophenotyping findings would most likely be seen in the neoplastic cells of monomorphic epitheliotropic intestinal T-cell lymphoma (formally type II enteropathy-associated T-cell lymphoma)?
    A. Large cells with angulated nuclei expressing CD103
    B. Large cells with anaplastic nuclei expressing ALK-1
    C. Small cells with round nuclei expressing CD34
    D. Small cells with round nuclei expressing CD8

27. A 50-year-old man presents with a one-year history of several large flat, erythematous lesions on his back and groin. Which of the following would be most suggestive of mycosis fungoides?
    A. Presence of similar lesions on the face and bilateral arms
    B. Presence of ulceration
    C. Detection of widespread lymphadenopathy
    D. Detection of several raised, indurated lesions in the same area

28. Which of the following histologic findings are most likely to be seen in a biopsy from a patient in the patch/plaque stage of mycosis fungoides?
    A. Dermal and perivascular infiltrate composed of small atypical lymphocytes with cerebriform nuclei showing focal epidermotropism and scattered Pautrier's microabscesses
    B. Dermal infiltrate composed of large lymphocytes with anaplastic, "horseshoe"-shaped nuclei, vesicular chromatin and prominent nucleoli
    C. Dermal infiltrate composed of small atypical lymphocytes at the dermal-epidermal border with focal epidermotropism, prominent epidermal spongiosis and scattered apoptotic keratinocytes
    D. Dermal infiltrate composed of large lymphocytes with round nuclei, dispersed chromatin, prominent nucleoli and a prominent "Grenz Zone"

29. Which of the following morphologic and immunophenotypic findings would be expected in the plaque stage of mycosis fungoides?
    A. Small atypical lymphocytes with irregular nuclei; CD2+, CD3+, CD4+, CD5+, CD7+, CD8+, CD26+, TCL-1+
    B. Large atypical cells with anaplastic, horseshoe-shaped nuclei; CD2-, CD3+, CD4+, CD5-, CD7-, CD8-, TIA-1+, CD30+
    C. Small atypical cells with irregular nuclei; CD2-, CD3+, CD4+, CD5+, CD7-, CD8-, CD25+, FOXP3+

D. Intermediate to large-sized atypical lymphocytes with irregular nuclei; CD2+, CD3+, CD4+, CD5-, CD7-, CD8-, CD26-, CD103-

30. Which of the following is associated with a worsened prognosis in mycosis fungoides?
   A. Presence of patches and plaques, involving <10% of total body surface area
   B. Presence of one or more tumors, ≥ 1.0 cm
   C. Expression of CD8 in the neoplastic cells
   D. Expression of CD4 in the neoplastic cells

31. Which of the following variants of mycosis fungoides is associated with a worsened prognosis?
   A. Folliculotropic mycosis fungoides
   B. Pagetoid reticulosis
   C. Granulomatous slack skin
   D. Hypopigmented mycosis fungoides

32. Which of the following variants of mycosis fungoides shows the *least* amount of epidermotropism?
   A. Folliculotropic mycosis fungoides
   B. Pagetoid reticulosis
   C. Granulomatous slack skin
   D. Hypopigmented mycosis fungoides

33. Which of the following is *not* usually seen in granulomatous slack skin?
   A. Involvement of the axilla and groin
   B. Numerous granulomas containing multi-nucleated giant cells
   C. Older age of onset compared to conventional mycosis fungoides
   D. Destruction of elastic fibers (elastolysis)

34. Which of the following would *not* be expected in pagetoid reticulosis?
   A. Extensive epidermotropism of the neoplastic infiltrate
   B. Expression of CD30 by the neoplastic cells
   C. An overall good prognosis
   D. Widespread dissemination at diagnosis

35. Which of the following is *least* likely to be seen in Sézary syndrome?
   A. Peripheral blood involvement by atypical lymphocytes with "cerebriform" nuclei accounting for >1000/μL of peripheral blood lymphocytes
   B. Prominent epidermotropism

C. Diffuse lymph node involvement
D. Erythroderma with hyperkeratosis of the palms and soles

36. What is the most common primary cutaneous lymphoma?
   A. Mycosis fungoides
   B. Primary cutaneous anaplastic large cell lymphoma
   C. Primary cutaneous follicle center lymphoma
   D. Primary cutaneous diffuse large B-cell lymphoma, leg type

37. Which of the following histologic findings would *not* be expected in a biopsy of subcutaneous panniculitis-like T-cell lymphoma?
   A. Dense infiltration of the subcutaneous adipose tissue
   B. Marked epidermotropism
   C. Fat necrosis
   D. Numerous histiocytes containing apoptotic debris

38. Which of the following immunophenotypic findings would *not* be expected in a biopsy of subcutaneous panniculitis-like T-cell lymphoma?
   A. Expression of CD4 by the neoplastic cells
   B. Expression of CD8 by the neoplastic cells
   C. Expression of TCR-αβ by the neoplastic cells
   D. Expression of granzyme B by the neoplastic cells

39. A 35-year-old man presents with several nodules on the chest and bilateral extremities. A biopsy of one of the nodules shows a lymphocytic infiltrate in the subcutaneous adipose tissue. The infiltrate contains numerous plasma cells, histiocytes, apoptotic debris, fat necrosis and several follicles with reactive germinal centers. Which of the following findings would *not* be expected?
   A. Degeneration of keratinocytes in the basal layer of the epidermis
   B. Prominent "rimming" of adipocytes by the lymphocytes
   C. Expression of CD8 by the lymphocytes
   D. Loss of CD7 expression by the lymphocytes

40. Which of the following is a characteristic finding in primary cutaneous CD4-positive small/medium T-cell lymphoproliferative disorder
   A. An aggressive clinical course

B. Presence of multiple lesions in the groin and buttocks

C. Expression of PD-1 by the neoplastic cells

D. Expression of CD30 by the neoplastic cells

41. Which of the following findings would *not* be expected in a patient with primary cutaneous CD8-positive aggressive epidermotropic cytotoxic T-cell lymphoma?

A. Sudden onset of numerous nodules with prominent ulceration

B. Expression of TCR-αβ by the neoplastic cells

C. Presence of visceral organ dissemination at diagnosis

D. Expression of EBV-encoded RNA by the neoplastic cells

42. A 45-year-old man presents with a 3-week history of numerous ulcerating papules and nodules on his chest and bilateral upper arms. Biopsy of one of the lesions shows a dense dermal infiltrate composed of large atypical lymphocytes with anaplastic, horseshoe-shaped nuclei that are positive for CD3, CD4 and CD30. When the patient returns to clinic two weeks later, the majority of lesions have disappeared. What is the most likely diagnosis?

A. Primary cutaneous anaplastic large cell lymphoma

B. Mycosis fungoides with large cell transformation

C. Lymphomatoid papulosis

D. Lymphomatous polyposis

43. A 45-year-old man presents with a 3-week history of numerous ulcerating papules and nodules on his chest and bilateral upper arms. Biopsy of one of the lesions shows a dense dermal infiltrate composed of large atypical lymphocytes with anaplastic, horseshoe-shaped nuclei that are positive for CD3, CD4 and CD30. When the patient returns to clinic two weeks later, the majority of lesions have disappeared. What is the most likely diagnosis?

A. Lymphomatoid papulosis, Type A

B. Lymphomatoid papulosis, Type B

C. Lymphomatoid papulosis, Type C

D. Lymphomatoid papulosis, Type D

44. Which of the following is seen in primary cutaneous anaplastic large cell lymphoma?

A. Translocation of the *ALK* gene

B. Strong expression of CD30 by the majority of neoplastic cells

C. Widespread dissemination at diagnosis

D. Presence of marked epidermotropism

45. What is the most common location of extranodal NK/T-cell lymphoma?

A. The skin

B. The gastrointestinal tract

C. The peripheral blood

D. The nasal cavity

46. Which of the following statements about extranodal NK/T-cell lymphoma is the most accurate?

A. This disease is most commonly seen in patients of European descent

B. This disease is highly associated with HHV-8 infection

C. This disease is commonly seen in patients of Asian descent

D. This disease is most commonly seen in pediatric patients

47. Which of the following morphologic findings is characteristic of extranodal NK/T-cell lymphoma?

A. Angiodestruction

B. Monomorphic tumor cell infiltrate

C. Minimal or complete lack of necrosis

D. Preservation of mucosal glands and overlying epithelium

48. Which of the following immunophenotypic findings is seen in extranodal NK/T-cell lymphoma?

A. Expression of TdT by the neoplastic cells

B. Expression of CD57 by the neoplastic cells

C. Expression of CD56 by the neoplastic cells

D. Expression of CD30 by the neoplastic cells

49. A 30-year-old Asian man presents with a recent history of fever, night sweats and 10-lb weight loss. Physical examination is negative for skin lesions but shows prominent splenomegaly. Imaging studies confirm the presence of splenomegaly; however, no lymphadenopathy is identified. Review of the complete blood count and peripheral blood smear shows pancytopenia with numerous large granular lymphocytes, some of

which are large with prominent nucleoli. Serologic studies for HIV and HTLV-1 are negative but serology for EBV is positive. Which of the following would be the most likely diagnosis?

A. Adult T-cell leukemia/lymphoma

B. T-cell large granular lymphocytic leukemia

C. Chronic lymphoproliferative disorder of NK-cells

D. Aggressive NK-cell leukemia

50. Which of the following is *not* frequently associated with angioimmunoblastic T-cell lymphoma?

A. Bilateral pleural effusions

B. Disseminated intravascular coagulation

C. Skin rash

D. Polyclonal hypergammaglobulinemia

51. Which of the following statements about angioimmunoblastic T-cell lymphoma is the most accurate?

A. Infectious disease is *not* a common complication of disease

B. The neoplastic T-cells are frequently infected with EBV

C. Most patients present with localized disease

D. Some patients may develop a secondary EBV-positive B-cell lymphoma

52. Which of the following morphologic findings is *not* typically seen in a lymph node involved by angioimmunoblastic T-cell lymphoma?

A. A prominent sinusoidal distribution of neoplastic cells

B. Expansion of high endothelial venules

C. Atypical small to intermediate-sized T-cells with abundant clear cytoplasm

D. Expanded follicular dendritic cell meshworks

53. Which of the following morphologic findings is typically seen in "Pattern II" of angioimmunoblastic T-cell lymphoma?

A. Preserved lymph node architecture, paracortical expansion and hyperplastic follicles

B. Effacement of lymph node architecture, paracortical expansion and numerous small, atretic follicles with "burned-out" germinal centers

C. Effacement of lymph node architecture, paracortical expansion and hyperplastic follicles

D. Effacement of lymph node architecture, paracortical expansion and lack of follicles

54. Which of the following statements regarding the immunophenotype of angioimmunoblastic T-cell lymphoma is correct?

A. The neoplastic cells have a follicular helper T-cell immunophenotype

B. The neoplastic cells have a cytotoxic T-cell immunophenotype

C. The neoplastic cells have a regulatory T-cell immunophenotype

D. The neoplastic T-cells are positive for EBV-encoded RNA (EBER)

55. Which of the following morphologic findings is most suggestive of ALK-positive anaplastic large cell lymphoma?

A. Presence of large lymphoid cells with abundant cytoplasm, bi-nucleation, and presence of prominent macronucleoli

B. Presence of large lymphoid cells with polylobated nuclei resembling the petals of a flower

C. Presence of large lymphoid cells with abundant cytoplasm, round nuclei, vesicular chromatin and numerous small nucleoli

D. Presence of large lymphoid cells with abundant cytoplasm and anaplastic, horseshoe-shaped nuclei

56. Of the immunohistochemical stains listed below, expression of which of the following would be most diagnostic of ALK-positive anaplastic large cell lymphoma?

A. Expression of EMA by the neoplastic cells

B. Expression of CD15 by the neoplastic cells

C. Expression of CD30 by the neoplastic cells

D. Expression of CD3 by the neoplastic cells

57. Which of the following statements regarding ALK-negative anaplastic large cell lymphoma is correct?

A. ALK-negative disease has a worse prognosis compared to ALK-positive disease

B. ALK-negative disease presents at a younger median age than ALK-positive disease

C. ALK-negative disease is negative for CD30

D. ALK-negative disease lacks the presence of hallmark cells

58. A lymph node biopsy shows near-total effacement by an infiltrate composed of numerous large cells with anaplastic, horseshoe-shaped nuclei. The large cells are positive for CD2, CD30 and TIA-1. Immunohistochemical stain for ALK shows positive staining in the nuclear, nucleolar and cytoplasmic regions of the neoplastic cells. Which of the following statements regarding this case is correct?
    A. Molecular genetic studies will show the presence of t(2;5)(p23;q35)
    B. Molecular genetic studies will show the presence of t(1;2)(q25;p23)
    C. Molecular genetic studies will show the presence of inv(2)(p23q35)
    D. Molecular genetic studies will demonstrate germline arrangement of the *TCR* gene

59. Which of the following statements regarding the prognosis of ALK-positive anaplastic large cell lymphoma is most correct?
    A. Most patients present with advanced stage disease and the prognosis is poor
    B. Most patients present with advanced stage disease and the prognosis is good
    C. Relapse almost never occurs
    D. Relapse occurs in some cases and is associated with chemo resistance and poor prognosis

60. A 47-year-old woman presents with swelling and pain around the left breast. She received bilateral breast implants approximately five years ago after undergoing mastectomy for invasive ductal carcinoma. Imaging studies show a large seroma surrounded by thickened capsule in the left breast. The effusion fluid and capsulectomy specimen shows numerous large atypical cells with irregular, anaplastic nuclei, including occasional cells with horseshoe-shaped nuclei. Which of the following immunohistochemical stains would be most useful in diagnosis?
    A. CD2
    B. CD15
    C. CD30
    D. ALK

61. Which of the following statements regarding breast implant-associated anaplastic large cell lymphoma is most correct?
    A. The disease is usually fatal

B. The presence of an effusion without a distinct mass is associated with a more aggressive clinical course
C. The disease occurs only with silicone-based implants
D. The presence of an effusion with a distinct mass is associated with a more aggressive clinical course

62. A 42-year-old man presents with a 2-month history of night sweats, weight loss and fever. Biopsy of a cervical lymph node shows near-complete effacement by a population of intermediate-sized atypical lymphocytes with round to irregular nuclei and clear cytoplasm. Flow cytometry and immunohistochemical studies show that the neoplastic cells are positive for CD2, CD3 and CD4. They are negative for CD5, CD7, CD8, CD10, CD20, CD25, CD26, CD30, CD34, CD56, PD-1, TCL-1 and ALK. Which of the following is the most appropriate diagnosis?
    A. Anaplastic large cell lymphoma, ALK-negative
    B. Angioimmunoblastic T-cell lymphoma
    C. Peripheral T-cell lymphoma, not otherwise specified
    D. Adult T-cell leukemia/lymphoma

63. Which of the following findings would *not* be seen in peripheral T-cell lymphoma, not otherwise specified?
    A. Intermediate-sized atypical lymphocytes admixed with an inflammatory infiltrate composed of eosinophils, histiocytes and plasma cells
    B. Large anaplastic cells with prominent nucleoli, positive for ALK
    C. Small cells with slightly irregular nuclei admixed with larger cells displaying Hodgkin/Reed-Sternberg-like morphology
    D. Large anaplastic cells with prominent nucleoli, weakly positive for CD30

64. Which of the following flow cytometry findings would be *least* useful in making a diagnosis of peripheral T-cell lymphoma, not otherwise specified?
    A. Dim CD3 expression
    B. Complete loss of CD7 expression
    C. Presence of CD10 expression
    D. Presence of HLA-DR expression

Answers to Chapter 6

1. B	17. D	33. C	49. D
2. C	18. D	34. D	50. B
3. D	19. B	35. B	51. D
4. B	20. D	36. A	52. A
5. C	21. B	37. B	53. B
6. A	22. A	38. A	54. A
7. B	23. D	39. B	55. D
8. A	24. C	40. C	56. C
9. D	25. A	41. D	57. A
10. C	26. D	42. C	58. A
11. D	27. D	43. C	59. B
12. B	28. A	44. B	60. C
13. C	29. D	45. D	61. D
14. D	30. B	46. C	62. C
15. B	31. A	47. A	63. B
16. B	32. A	48. C	64. D

Answers to Chapter 6 (with Explanations)

1. B

The overall findings are most consistent with T-cell large granular lymphocytic leukemia (T-LGLL). T-LGLL is characterized by a persistent (> six months) clonal proliferation of T-cell large granular lymphocytes (LGLs) in the peripheral blood. The LGLs show characteristic morphology: abundant basophilic cytoplasm containing large, reddish-pink (azurophilic) granules, round to slightly irregular nuclei and condensed chromatin without nucleoli. Using electron microscopy, it can be seen that the azurophilic granules are composed of numerous perpendicularly arranged microtubules referred to as parallel tubular arrays.

T-LGLL is most commonly seen in older men and woman (50–60 years old) and has an indolent clinical course characterized by cytopenias (most commonly neutropenia and anemia), bone marrow involvement, mild splenomegaly, autoimmune symptoms and symptoms related to cytopenias (such as recurrent infections due to neutropenia). The other choices listed also have distinct morphologic findings and tend to show a more aggressive clinical course.

2. C

Large granular lymphocytic leukemia may result from a clonal proliferation of either cytotoxic T-cells (CTC) or natural killer (NK) cells. Both types of disease show similar clinicopathologic features, including a characteristic interstitial and intrasinusoidal pattern of bone marrow infiltration, but are classified separately as "T-cell large granular lymphocytic leukemia" (T-LGLL) and "Chronic lymphoproliferative disorder of NK-cells" (CLPD-NK), respectively. The two types cannot be distinguished by morphology but can be differentiated by immunophenotype.

T-LGLL has a CTC immunophenotype: CD2+, CD3+, CD4- and CD5 +/-, CD7 +/-, CD8+, CD16+, CD56-, CD57+ and CD94+.

CLPD-NK has an NK-cell immunophenotype: CD2+, CD3-, CD4-, CD5+/-, CD7+/-, CD8+, CD16+, CD56+, CD57-, CD94+.

In general, CTC can be thought of as CD3+, CD8+, CD57+ and NK-cells can be thought of as CD3-, CD8+, CD56+. However, it is important to note that T-cell lymphoproliferative disorders are characterized by variable loss or gain of antigen expression (such as aberrant expression of CD56 in T-LGLL). Antigens such as CD2, CD3, CD5 and CD7 frequently show aberrant negative/dim or bright staining. As such, accurate diagnosis requires correlation with clinical history and molecular genetic studies.

3. D

As mentioned, CTC and NK-cells show distinct but potentially overlapping immunophenotypic features. Thus, the most reliable method of differentiation is evaluation of the *TCR* gene by either PCR or Southern Blot analysis. Unlike cytotoxic T-cells, NK-cells retain a germline configuration of the *TCR* gene during their development. Thus, a lack of *TCR*-γ and *TCR*-β gene rearrangement (germline configuration) by PCR is one of the most reliable methods of distinguishing NK-cells from CTCs. In the above scenario, the presence of a monoclonal rearrangement of the *TCR*-β and/or *TCR*-γ gene would be suggestive of T-LGLL. Expression of TCR αβ by flow cytometry is most commonly seen in T-LGLL; however, rare cases with expression of TCR γδ are also seen. It is also important to note that PCR analysis of the *TCR* gene *does not* correlate with the type of TCR molecule expressed on the surface of the cell and should not be used to classify the type of T-cell (αβ versus γδ). However, this information can be obtained through flow cytometry studies as mentioned earlier.

4. B

Natural killer cells, being part of the innate immune system, utilize antibody-independent, major histocompatibility complex–unrestricted cytotoxicity that is mediated by cytotoxic molecules (e.g., perforin, granzyme B, TIA-1) and regulated by activating and inhibiting NK-cell receptors such as the CD94/NKG2 family of receptors. As such, they do not rearrange the *TCR* gene or express the T-cell receptor (TCR) on their surface. This results in the failure of the "TCR-complex" (TCR plus two CD3ε chains, one CD3γ chain, one CD3δ chain and a zeta homodimer) to form on the cell surface. It is important to note, however, that natural killer cells can show cytoplasmic expression of epsilon and zeta chains. Although this does not equate to a full CD3 molecule, many immunohistochemical stains may react with the cytoplasmic CD3 epsilon chains and give a positive result. However, flow cytometry will be negative for surface CD3. Of note, NK-cells are positive for cytoplasmic CD3 (cCD3), which can be detected by flow cytometry. In addition, NK-cells show expression of CD2, CD16 and CD56. CD56 is an isoform of neural cell adhesion molecule (N-CAM) and is a very sensitive (but not specific) marker for NK-cells.

5. C

Although the clinical course of T-cell large granular lymphocytic leukemia (T-LGLL) is generally indolent, many patients will be symptomatic at diagnosis. Patients experience a mixture of both hematologic and autoimmune disease manifestations. The hematologic manifestations primarily involve cytopenias as well as infiltration of the bone marrow, spleen and liver. Infiltration of these organs tends to be mild. Mild lymphadenopathy may be seen but the presence of diffuse areas of lymphadenopathy would be highly atypical. Neutropenia and anemia are the most commonly seen cytopenias; thrombocytopenia is less frequent but is occasionally seen. Cytopenias are a major source of morbidity and mortality. For example, recurrent bacterial infections due to neutropenia can be seen and can range from mild skin infections to, infrequently, fatal sepsis. In addition, severe anemia due to pure red cell aplasia can be seen in a subset of patients, especially those of Asian descent. Autoimmune manifestations are very common in T-LGLL; a large percentage of patients will have detectable Rheumatoid factor, antinuclear antibodies and polyclonal hypergammaglobulinemia.

6. A

T-cell large granular lymphocytic leukemia (T-LGLL) is frequently reported in patients with autoimmune disease, most commonly Rheumatoid arthritis (RA) and Felty's syndrome (characterized by the combined presence of Rheumatoid arthritis, splenomegaly and neutropenia). Patients with T-LGLL and RA or Felty's syndrome have a high frequency of human leukocyte antigen (HLA)-DR4. In addition, T-LGLL can be accompany numerous other conditions including B-cell lymphoproliferative disorders (most frequently chronic lymphocytic leukemia), myelodysplastic syndrome and following bone marrow or solid organ transplant. HTLV-1 infection is more commonly seen in patients with adult T-cell leukemia/lymphoma (ATLL).

7. B

A subset of mature T-cell neoplasms is characterized by sudden onset of aggressive disease with peripheral blood involvement and widespread dissemination at presentation. Unfortunately, these disorders may show overlapping clinicopathologic features and a broad differential diagnosis with judicious use of ancillary studies is needed for accurate diagnosis. Of the choices listed, only T-cell large granular lymphocytic leukemia (T-LGLL) would not be considered in the differential diagnosis as it is associated with a chronic indolent course. The remaining choices are likely to show an aggressive clinical course with disseminated disease including leukemic involvement and skin involvement. However, Sézary syndrome is most often encountered as a late complication of mycosis fungoides and is unlikely to present with such a sudden onset. Adult T-cell leukemia/lymphoma (ATLL) is caused by HTLV-1 infection and is seen in patients from regions where the virus is endemic such as Japan, Central Africa and certain parts of Central and South America. Thus, the most likely diagnosis is T-cell prolymphocytic leukemia (T-PLL). In addition to the presence of aggressive, disseminated disease, T-PLL is associated with marked leukocytosis, often >100 x 10^9/L.

8. A

The majority of patients with T-cell prolymphocytic leukemia will present with leukemic involvement characterized by the presence of medium-sized atypical lymphocytes with round to irregular nuclei, condensed chromatin and a large prominent single nucleolus. The chromatin surrounding the nucleolus is very condensed, giving it a "punched out" appearance. The cytoplasm is deeply basophilic, does not contain granules and may show cytoplasmic projections or "blebs." In contrast, the leukemic cells in patients with adult T-cell leukemia/lymphoma show hypercondensed/hyperchromatic nuclei with a polylobated shape that resembles the petals of a flower, often referred to as "flower cells." The leukemic cells in patients with mycosis fungoides/Sézary syndrome also contain irregular nuclei with numerous lobulations, which resemble the gyri of the brain, often referred to as "cerebriform" morphology. Of note, approximately 20% of patients with T-prolymphocytic leukemia will have leukemic cells that are small and without prominent nucleoli (small cell variant). Furthermore, heterogeneous and potentially overlapping morphology has been reported for the leukemic cells in all of the above-mentioned conditions. As such, additional ancillary studies are necessary for accurate diagnosis.

9. D

In most patients with T-cell prolymphocytic leukemia (T-PLL), the bone marrow architecture is effaced by diffuse sheets of atypical lymphocytes. The typical prolymphocyte morphology is less conspicuous in these samples and is better appreciated in peripheral blood smears. The cells in the infiltrate show increased expression of the oncoprotein TCL1, which can be visualized by immunohistochemistry.

10. C

T-cell prolymphocytic leukemia (T-PLL) shows a mature, post-thymic immunophenotype. Unlike other T-cell lymphoproliferative disorders which tend to show loss or diminished intensity of T-cell markers, T-PLL shows expression of pan T-cell markers such as CD2, CD5 and CD7 with frequent bright CD7 expression. Cytoplasmic expression of CD3 is present, but surface expression of CD3 may be dim or absent in a subset of cases. The majority of cases are positive for CD4; however, approximately 25% of cases show co-expression of CD4 and CD8, and the minority of cases (approximately 15%) are positive for CD8. The neoplastic cells are positive for TCRα/β and there is no expression of cytotoxic markers such as CD56 or CD57 or immaturity

markers such as TdT, CD34, or CD1a. They are positive for CD26, which is useful in diagnosis and as a therapeutic target. They also strongly express CD52, which is similarly useful in treatment. The anti-CD52 monoclonal antibody alemtuzumab is frequently used in combination with chemotherapy. In general, T-PLL can be considered to have the following immunophenotype: CD1a-, CD2+, cytoplasmic CD3+, surface CD3+/-, CD5+, CD7+ (bright); CD26+ CD56-, CD57-, TCRαβ+, TDT- and in order of *decreasing* frequency: CD4+/CD8-, CD4+/CD8+, CD4-/CD8+

11. D

Numerous genetic abnormalities have been associated with T-cell prolymphocytic leukemia (T-PLL). The most frequent abnormalities involve inversions or translocations in chromosome 14 such as inv(14)(q11q32), t(14;14)(q11q32). These rearrangements result in juxtaposition of the *TCRA/D* gene at 14q11 with the *TCL-1* and *TCL1b* genes on 14q32. A smaller subset of cases have t(X;14)(q28q11). This results in juxtaposition of the *TCRA/D* gene with the *MTCP1* gene on chromosome Xq28. *TCL1*, *TCL1-b* and *MTCP1* are essentially homologous and juxtaposition of these genes with the *TCRA/D* gene results in their activation and overexpression which ultimately results in overexpression of the TCL1 protein. Detection of this protein by immunohistochemical studies is useful in diagnosis. TCL1 binds to and enhances activity of the AKT1 kinase and promotes its transportation into the nucleus. The overall effect is increased cell proliferation and survival. Other common genetic abnormalities in T-PLL include abnormalities of chromosome 8, including gains of 8q, which lead to increased copies of the oncogene *MYC*, and deletion/loss of the Ataxia Telangiectasia Mutated (*ATM*) gene on chromosome 11q23. In contrast, isochrome 7q is highly associated with hepatosplenic T-cell lymphoma.

12. B

The causal relationship between T-cell prolymphocytic leukemia (T-PLL) and the retrovirus HTLV-1 has been discussed, although it is important to recognize that the infection alone is insufficient for leukemogenesis and that HTLV-1 infection causes other nonmalignant disorders. In addition, there is a long latency between infection (most often in childhood) and development of disease. Nevertheless, serologic or molecular genetic-based detection of the virus is a useful means of diagnosis. Similar to another retrovirus, HIV, HTLV-1 infects CD4+ T-cells and shows similar modes of transmission including blood product administration, intravenous drug abuse, mother to infant transmission (especially through breastfeeding) and sexual transmission. The virus integrates its genome into the host cell and causes transcription of numerous viral proteins including the TAX protein which promotes proliferation via numerous mechanisms including stimulation of T-cell growth, inhibition of apoptosis, disruption of DNA and activation of several signal transduction pathways. Interestingly, many patients with T-PLL also have an associated T-cell immunodeficiency and their clinical course may be complicated by opportunistic infections such *Pneumocystis jiroveci*, *Stronglyoides stercorlais*, as well as viral disease/reactivation such CMV, HSV and VZV. The cause of this immunodeficiency is incompletely understood but the CD3+/CD4+/CD25+, TCR αβ+ immunophenotype seen in T-PLL is also seen in regulatory T-cells (Treg), suggesting that T-PLL is derived from this cell type, whose main function is immune suppression. This notion is supported by the expression of FOXP3 protein in a subset of cases. This protein is a key regulator in the development and function of regulatory T-cells.

13. C

Patients with acute adult T-cell leukemia/lymphoma typically present with peripheral blood lymphocytosis and eosinophilia. Hypercalcemia with lytic bone lesions is a very common and characteristic finding. Most cases present with widespread dissemination and tumor burden which can be manifested by an increased serum lactate dehydrogenase (LDH) level.

14. D

Although previously mentioned extranodal sites may be involved by adult T-cell leukemia/lymphoma, the skin is the most frequently involved extranodal site of disease, being seen in approximately 50% of patients. Skin involvement can be seen in all four variants of the disease: acute, lymphomatous, chronic and smoldering and is typically heterogeneous, ranging from exfoliating rashes to papules and large nodules with ulceration. The skin lesions are also histologically

diverse but frequently show a dermal and perivascular infiltrate with occasional epidermotropism and formation of Pautrier-like abscesses, mimicking mycosis fungoides. The cellular morphology is highly variable, ranging from small cells with minimal cytologic atypia to larger cells with cerebriform-like nuclei. This variability in morphology and propensity for morphologic overlap with other types of cutaneous T-cell lymphoma necessitates strong clinical correlation and use of ancillary techniques for accurate diagnosis.

15. B

There are four variants of adult T-cell leukemia/lymphoma. The most common type, the acute, leukemic variant, is characterized by peripheral blood involvement by neoplastic cells with characteristic "flower cell" morphology. This variant shows widespread disease dissemination at presentation with hypercalcemia, lytic lesions, elevated LDH, lymphadenopathy and extranodal disease in the skin, liver and spleen. Occasionally disease may be seen in the GI tract, respiratory tract and central nervous system. Cardiac involvement can occur as a terminal event.

The lymphomatous variant is the most frequently encountered variant in the Western hemisphere. As the name implies, this variant is characterized by nodal involvement without peripheral blood involvement. This is analogous to the separation of chronic lymphocytic leukemia and small lymphocytic lymphoma by primarily leukemic versus primarily nodal disease. The lymphomatous variant also shows widespread disease dissemination with frequent cutaneous involvement and an aggressive clinical course. A subset of patient will eventually progress to the acute, leukemic form of disease. Both the acute and lymphomatous variant have a poor prognosis with median survival of less than one year.

The chronic variant has a more heterogeneous presentation and clinical course. Patients typically have cutaneous involvement in the form of an exfoliative skin rash, but without leukemic involvement. Patients may have absolute lymphocytosis and show rare atypical lymphocytes. The detection of flower cells in the peripheral blood of these patients is considered a poor prognostic sign. Hypercalcemia and widespread disease are not common but a subset of patients may show hepatosplenomegaly. Most patients can be expected to have a median survival of two years but a subset (approximately 25%) may eventually transform to the acute variant.

The smoldering variant of adult T-cell leukemia/lymphoma has the most indolent clinical course with an expected median survival of greater than two years. These patients typically present with disease limited to the skin, without nodal, peripheral blood or extranodal involvement.

16. **B**

Adult T-cell leukemia/lymphoma is frequently positive for CD3, CD4 and CD25. CD25 is the interleukin-2 receptor (IL-2), and is a potential therapeutic target. As mentioned, the neoplastic cells are believed to be derived from regulatory T-cells. As such, the expression of CCR4 (chemokine receptor 4) and FOXP3 can be seen in a subset of cases and may aid in diagnosis. Co-expression of CD4 and CD8 may rarely be seen in adult T-cell leukemia/lymphoma but is more commonly associated with T-prolymphocytic leukemia, as is the expression of TCL-1.

17. **D**

Lymph node involvement by adult T-cell leukemia/lymphoma shows a wide array of morphologic features.

The most common appearance has been termed the pleomorphic (medium and large cell type) variant of disease and is characterized by the presence of medium and large-sized atypical lymphocytes with highly irregular nuclear contours. The nuclear irregularity ranges from mild to anaplastic and it is not uncommon to see large cells with "bizarre" nuclei, cerebriform nuclei or cells with Hodgkin/Reed-Sternberg-like morphology.

The pleomorphic small cell type shows a proliferation of small lymphocytes with minimal nuclear atypia.

The anaplastic large cell type shows a uniform proliferation of large atypical cells with abundant cytoplasm, anaplastic nuclei and occasional nucleoli. These cells greatly resemble those seen in anaplastic large cell lymphoma (ALCL) and diagnosis would require extensive use of ancillary studies. Nevertheless, ALCL is characterized by the presence of intrasinusoidal and subcapsular infiltrate that mimics the pattern of infiltration seen in metastatic carcinoma.

A rare Hodgkin-like variant has been described which is characterized by the presence of preserved lymph node architecture with paracortical expansion by a proliferation of small to medium atypical lymphocytes admixed with large cells showing Hodgkin/Reed Sternberg-like morphology. The Hodgkin/Reed-Sternberg-like cells express CD15 and CD30 and are positive for EBV-encoded RNA (EBER). This variant is felt to be a precursor lesion to overt disease.

A rare variant that resembles angioimmunoblastic T-cell lymphoma (AITL) has also been described. This variant shows all the characteristic features of AITL, including a proliferation of small to medium-sized atypical lymphocytes with abundant, clear cytoplasm admixed eosinophils and plasma cells associated with proliferation of high endothelial venules.

18. **D**

Although a monoclonal rearrangement of the *TCR* gene and a complex karyotype are frequently detected in the neoplastic cells of patients with adult T-cell leukemia/lymphoma, they are not entirely specific. As mentioned, development of adult T-cell leukemia/lymphoma is preceded by infection with the HTLV-1 virus. Evidence of infection by serologic detection of antibodies against the virus, supports the diagnosis.

Detection of integration of proviral HTLV-1 DNA in the clonal cells is a very specific method of diagnosis. The viral DNA encodes numerous proteins such as the TAX protein. Recently, another virally encoded gene known as the HTLV-1 basic leucine zipper factor (*HBZ*) has been consistently found in the neoplastic cells of the disease and likely plays a large role in oncogenesis. Detection of *HBZ* expression may be another useful method of diagnosis.

19. **B**

Despite the frequent presence of widespread disease dissemination at presentation, the bone marrow in patients with adult T-cell leukemia/lymphoma is frequently negative or only minimally involved. This is true even in cases with marked peripheral blood lymphocytosis.

20. **D**

Hepatosplenic T-cell lymphoma is a rare disorder that is frequently seen in young patients and shows a male predominance. The patients typically have a history of immunologic disease, and can be seen in patients who are receiving immunosuppressive therapy for solid organ transplantation. Other associated immunologic conditions include inflammatory bowel disease, malaria and pregnancy. Most patients present with B-type symptoms, hepatosplenomegaly and cytopenias (most frequently thrombocytopenia). Widespread disease, lymphadenopathy, and peripheral blood involvement are rare. Nevertheless, most patients have bone marrow involvement at presentation. The neoplastic cells have a characteristic intrasinusoidal pattern of infiltration in the bone marrow.

21. B

Hepatosplenic T-cell lymphoma frequently involves the bone marrow and shows a characteristic intrasinusoidal infiltrate that is composed of small- to medium-sized lymphocytes with minimal cytologic atypia. As such, the infiltrate is hard to appreciate on hematoxylin and eosin-stained core biopsy specimens and recognition is greatly aided by immunohistochemistry.

Hepatosplenic T-cell lymphoma shows an immunophenotype similar to nonactivated cytotoxic γδ T-cells. In general, the immunophenotype is CD2+, CD3+, CD5-, CD7+/-, and frequently CD4-/CD8-. Rare cases are CD4-/CD8+. CD16 and CD56 may be expressed but CD57 is frequently negative. Immaturity markers such as TDT and CD1a are negative.

Cytotoxic markers such as TIA-1, granzyme M and CD94 are positive. However, markers of activated cytotoxic T-cells, such as granzyme B and perforin, are frequently negative. Detection of TCR-γδ aids in diagnosis, but requires the use of flow cytometry. Of note, rare cases showing a TCR-αβ phenotype have been reported but appear to show similar clinicopathologic features to cases with a TCR-γδ phenotype.

22. A

Cytogenetic studies demonstrate the presence of isochrome 7q [i(7)(q10)] in most cases of hepatosplenic T-cell lymphoma. This structural abnormality results in partial trisomy of 7q. However, the presence of additional copies of isochrome 7q or 7q can be seen in some cases, and is often associated with disease progression. Furthermore, a

ring chromosome 7, which results in the amplification of 7q, may be rarely found. Thus, all of these abnormalities result in increased expression of genetic material from the long arm of chromosome 7. The significance of this chromosomal region and its relationship to the development of hepatosplenic T-cell lymphoma remains under investigation. Other abnormalities such as trisomy 8 and deletion/loss of chromosome Y may also be observed. Deletion of chromosome 7q is often seen in myelodysplastic syndrome.

23. D

Enteropathy-associated T-cell lymphoma (formally Type I enteropathy associated T-cell lymphoma) is associated with celiac disease (gluten-sensitive enteropathy). The diagnosis of celiac disease is often made concurrently or following a recent diagnosis of adult-onset celiac disease or dermatitis herpetiformis (cutaneous manifestation of celiac disease). Rare cases are found in older patients who were diagnosed with celiac disease in childhood. Most patients present with malabsorption (bulky diarrhea, weight loss, anemia, vitamin deficiency). Many patients present with abdominal pain secondary to intestinal perforation. The disease is most frequently found in the jejunum or ileum; however, multiple areas of involvement are frequently found at diagnosis.

24. C

Enteropathy-associated T-cell lymphoma (formally classified as Type I enteropathy-associated T-cell lymphoma) commonly presents as small, multifocal ulcerating mucosal nodules. However, the macroscopic appearance may range from very subtle mucosal changes to a large exophytic mass with extensive ulceration. The mesentery and mesenteric lymph nodes are very frequently involved and concomitant ulceration, fissures and strictures may also be present.

The microscopic appearance of enteropathy-associated T-cell lymphoma is variable. The infiltrate is generally quite extensive, extending from the mucosa through the wall and into the mesentery (transmural infiltrate). Commonly, there is extensive ulceration of the mucosa and the infiltrate is accompanied by a heavy inflammatory infiltrate and extensive necrosis. The inflammatory component may be heavy enough to partially obscure the neoplastic infiltrate.

The cells of the neoplastic infiltrate show pleomorphic morphology with medium to large cells with round to angulated nuclei, vesicular chromatin, prominent nucleoli and variable amounts of eosinophilic cytoplasm.

This is distinct from monomorphic epitheliotropic intestinal T-cell lymphoma (formally classified as Type II enteropathy-associated T-cell lymphoma), which is characterized by a monomorphic population of small to medium-sized cells with round nuclei, variably condensed chromatin and a rim of pale eosinophilic cytoplasm.

25. A

Because of their shared tendency for localization to the small bowel, enteropathy associated T-cell lymphoma and monomorphic epitheliotropic intestinal T-cell lymphoma were originally classified as variants of the same disease (Type I enteropathy associated T-cell lymphoma and Type II enteropathy associated T-cell lymphoma, respectively).

However, the two disease are distinct in almost every other aspect and are now viewed as separate diseases.

The neoplastic cells in enteropathy associated T-cell lymphoma are pleomorphic while the neoplastic cells in monomorphic epitheliotropic intestinal T-cell lymphoma are monomorphic. The neoplastic cells of each disease also have distinct immunophenotypes.

In addition, enteropathy associated T-cell lymphoma is associated with celiac disease and patients frequently have a HLADQA1*0501, DQB*0201 genotype.

26. D

The neoplastic cells of enteropathy associated T-cell lymphoma (formally Type I enteropathy associated T-cell lymphoma) are pleomorphic, medium to large-sized cells with round to angulated nuclei and vesicular chromatin. The neoplastic cells have an immunophenotype similar to intraepithelial T-cells. They are usually CD4-/CD8- and CD56- and are frequently CD3+, CD5-, CD7+ and CD103+ .

In contrast, the neoplastic cells of monomorphic epitheliotropic intestinal T-cell lymphoma (formally Type II enteropathy associated T-cell lymphoma) are monomorphic, small cells with round nuclei and clear cytoplasm. These cells frequently express CD8 and CD56.

27. D

The diagnosis of mycosis fungoides requires correlation of morphologic, immunophenotypic and, occasionally, molecular genetic data with both the clinical appearance and behavior of the associated lesions.

Mycosis fungoides typically occurs in older patients, who present with lesions in sun-protected areas of the body such as the back, buttocks, chest and groin. The disease is partially defined by the tendency of the lesions to progress through several stages. The initial, early lesions of the disease, referred to as patches, are round to oval, flat and erythematous and may show scale formation or hypopigmentation. These lesions may progress to form indurated, slightly raised lesions referred to as plaques. The plaques may progress to form raised, fungating lesions known as tumors. Plaques and tumors may show ulceration. At all stages, the lesions are usually multifocal and heterogeneous in size and shape (although rare unifocal cases have been reported). Nevertheless, the clinical course is predominantly indolent, with most patients remaining in the early stages of disease for several years. Widespread lymphadenopathy, distant metastasis and peripheral blood involvement may be seen in later stages of the disease but are uncommon in the early, patch stage.

28. A

The histologic features of mycosis fungoides vary with the clinical stage of disease. In the early patch stage, the histologic findings may be limited to a scant dermal and perivascular infiltrate of small lymphocytes with minimal atypia and little to no epidermotropism. In the late patch and plaque stage, there is a "bandlike" dermal infiltrate composed of small atypical lymphocytes with irregular, folded nuclei that resemble the gyri of the brain (cerebriform morphology). The atypical cells infiltrate into the overlying epidermis (epidermotropism) and may collect along the basal layer of the epidermis forming a "string of pearls"-like appearance. In addition, the atypical cells may form aggregates in the epidermis, referred to as "Pautrier's microabscesses."

As the lesion progresses to the tumor stage, there is a loss of epidermotropism and the dermal infiltrate becomes more dense and nodular. As the lesion progresses, there is an increased tendency for the atypical lymphocytes to become large with round nuclei, dispersed chromatin and prominent nucleoli (referred to as "transformed" lymphocytes). Infiltrates containing >25% transformed lymphocytes are diagnosed as mycosis fungoides with "large cell transformation" and are likely to have a more aggressive clinical course.

Biopsies of the tumor stage may contain a dermal infiltrate composed of large lymphocytes with no epidermotropism but would not be expected in the patch/plaque stage. Furthermore, the presence of a "Grenz Zone" (a layer of uninvolved dermis between the epidermis and the dermal infiltrate) is more often seen in cutaneous B-cell lymphomas. Finally, many inflammatory conditions can mimic the histologic appearance of mycosis fungoides. Clinical correlation is needed for diagnosis, but in general the presence of significant spongiosis, acute inflammation and destruction of the epidermis should prompt consideration of inflammatory disease.

29. D

The neoplastic cells of mycosis fungoides show a mature T-helper cell immunophenotype. They are frequently positive for CD3, CD4 and negative for CD8. A minority of cases, especially in pediatric patients, are CD4- and CD8+. The neoplastic cells frequently show aberrant loss of one or more pan T-cell markers such as CD2, CD5 and (most commonly) CD7. CD103 (αE integrin) is involved in localization of the neoplastic cells to the epithelium and is more frequently expressed in the late patch/early plaque stage when epidermotropism is more prominent. CD26 (dipeptidyl-aminopeptidase IV) is a membrane glycoprotein expressed on normal T-cells that is frequently lost in mycosis fungoides and the related Sézary syndrome.

30. B

Prognosis in mycosis fungoides is determined by clinical stage rather than morphology or immunophenotype. The recently revised clinical staging system for mycosis fungoides uses the TNMB system. The T stage is determined not only by the type of lesions present (patches, plaques or tumors) but also by the percentage of body surface area involvement. In general, the presence of patches and plaques involving ≥ 10% body surface area, the presence of one or more tumors and/or the presence of erythroderma involving ≥80% body surface area are associated with a higher clinical stage and worsened prognosis. The N stage is determined by the amount of lymph node involvement and by the detection of clonal TCR gene rearrangement by PCR. Similar to other staging systems, the M stage is determined by the absence or presence of visceral organ involvement. Finally, the B stage is determined by detection and enumeration of neoplastic lymphocytes in the peripheral blood. The presence of neoplastic cells >5% of peripheral blood lymphocytes and/or detection of monoclonal TCR gene rearrangement in the peripheral blood increases the stage. The presence of neoplastic cells >1000/µL in the peripheral blood is considered to be stage IV disease and is one of the criteria for diagnosis of Sézary syndrome.

Patients with Stage I to IIa are considered to have "limited stage disease" and show an overall survival measured in decades whereas patients with Stage IIb to IVb are considered to have "advanced stage disease" and have an overall survival of approximately 1–5 years.

31. A

There are several variants of mycosis fungoides that show distinct clinical, morphologic and prognostic features. Of the listed variants, only the folliculotropic variant has been associated with a worsened prognosis. This variant frequently presents as disseminated papules in the hair-bearing areas of the head and neck with possible alopecia of the involved areas. The neoplastic cells typically spare the epidermis and localize to the hair follicles of the skin. This is often accompanied by distention of the hair follicles by excess mucin production, referred to as follicular mucinosis. The deep localization of the disease makes the lesions less responsive to skin-targeted therapy, which may contribute to the worsened prognosis.

32. A

Folliculotropic mycosis fungoides infiltrates the hair follicles in the deep dermis, leaving the superficial dermis and overlying epidermis relatively uninvolved. Pagetoid reticulosis preferentially affects the extremities, especially the hands and feet. The atypical cells show marked epidermotropism (pagetoid distribution) and are often associated with epidermal hyperplasia and marked hyperkeratosis that imparts a verrucous or warty appearance to the associated lesions. There is typically little to no dermal involvement. This variant typically occurs in younger patients, infrequently disseminates and shows a good prognosis compared to conventional disease. Of note, this description applies only to the localized form of disease (also known as Woringer-Kolopp disease). The disseminated form, also known as Ketron-Goodman disease, has a much more aggressive clinical course and is felt to be a subtype of primary cutaneous aggressive epidermotropic CD8 positive cytotoxic T-cell lymphoma. Granulomatous slack skin heavily involves the papillary and deep dermis and can show variable amounts of epidermal involvement. Hypopigmented mycosis fungoides (named for the light color of the lesions) shows histologic features that are similar to conventional mycosis fungoides, including epidermotropism, but is more frequently associated with a younger age of onset, frequent expression of CD8 and a good prognosis.

33. C

Granulomatous slack skin is a rare variant of mycosis fungoides that occurs in young patients and commonly involves the axilla and groin. The infiltrate heavily involves the dermis and subcutaneous lobules and contains numerous granulomas composed of epithelioid histiocytes and multi-nucleated giant cells surrounded by small lymphocytes. The histiocytes appear to be responsible for the prominent destruction of elastic fibers (elastolysis) associated with the disease. Identification of the degenerated elastic fibers is aided by special stains and is useful in diagnosis. The loss of elastic fibers contributes to the development of large, pendulous skin folds in the affected area, leading to an appearance of loose or "slack" skin. Diagnosis is aided by microscopic examination of the superficial dermis and epidermis, which typically shows the morphologic and immunophenotypic findings of conventional mycosis fungoides. Of note, several types of lymphoma may contain variable amounts of

granulomatous inflammation and a "granulomatous" variant of mycosis fungoides has been described. However, this variant lacks the characteristic pendulous lesions and elastolysis of granulomatous slack skin and appears to be similar to conventional disease in other respects.

34. D

Pagetoid reticulosis is characterized by extensive epidermotropism (pagetoid distribution) of the neoplastic cells. By definition, the disease is localized and has a relatively good prognosis. The neoplastic cells are CD3+, CD4+, CD8- and CD30+. A subset of cases are CD4-, CD8+.

35. B

Sézary syndrome is defined by the triad of erythroderma, generalized lymphadenopathy and the detection of clonally related neoplastic T-cells in the skin, peripheral blood and lymph nodes. The neoplastic cells show morphologic and immunophenotypic features similar to mycosis fungoides including the presence of neoplastic cells with cerebriform nuclei referred to as Sézary cells. The disease is often preceded by mycosis fungoides and as such, Sézary syndrome can be thought of as the leukemic form of mycosis fungoides. Nevertheless, the neoplastic cells of mycosis fungoides and Sézary syndrome show immunophenotypic differences that indicate they are derived from different memory T-cell subsets. Erythroderma refers to the presence of diffusely red skin that is often pruritic with marked exfoliation that may be accompanied by palmoplantar hyperkeratosis. Despite this, biopsies may show minimal or nonspecific changes. However, a subset of patients will show histologic findings similar to those seen in the tumor stage of mycosis fungoides, with a dense dermal infiltrate composed of atypical lymphocytes and minimal to no epidermotropism. At diagnosis, there is generally widespread lymphadenopathy and involvement of visceral organs, including the heart, can be seen in advanced disease. An absolute Sézary cell count of at least 1000/μL in the peripheral blood is required for diagnosis.

36. A

Primary cutaneous lymphomas are those that arise in the skin and are limited to this location at diagnosis. Primary cutaneous lymphomas may show overlapping morphology with other systemic lymphomas, but have distinct clinico-pathologic features as well as separate classification and staging systems. Primary cutaneous T-cell lymphomas are far more common (approximately 70% of cases) than primary cutaneous B-cell lymphomas, and mycosis fungoides is the most common primary cutaneous lymphoma, accounting for approximately 40–60% of cases.

37. B

Subcutaneous panniculitis-like T-cell lymphoma is a rare primary cutaneous lymphoma that characteristically involves the subcutaneous adipose tissue with minimal to no involvement of the overlying dermis and epidermis. The infiltrate is composed of small to medium-sized atypical lymphocytes admixed with numerous histiocytes, which may contain apoptotic debris or show hemophagocytosis. There is often abundant tumor cell karyorrhexis and fat necrosis in the background. The presence of atypical cells encircling individual adipocytes, referred to as adipocyte rimming, is another characteristic morphologic finding.

38. A

Subcutaneous panniculitis-like T-cell lymphoma shows a mature, αβ cytotoxic T-cell immunophenotype. As such, they are CD3+, CD4- and CD8+ and express cytotoxic T-cell markers such as TIA-1, perforin and granzyme B. The neoplastic cells are negative for EBV-encoded RNA (EBER), CD30 and CD56. Of note, only cases with a TCR-αβ phenotype are classified as subcutaneous panniculitis-like T-cell lymphoma. Cases expressing a TCR-γδ phenotype are considered to be a variant of primary cutaneous γ-δ T-cell lymphoma.

39. B

Lupus-associated panniculitis (LEP), also known as lupus profundis, shows overlapping clinical and morphologic features with subcutaneous panniculitis-like T-cell lymphoma. Differentiation between these two conditions is challenging, and diagnosis requires close correlation with clinical and laboratory findings. Both conditions show a lymphoid infiltrate in the subcutaneous adipose tissue with variable degrees of cytologic atypia, numerous histiocytes, abundant karyorrhexis and fat necrosis. However, certain morphologic features, such as the presence of epidermal atrophy, degeneration of basal keratinocytes, plasma cells

and reactive follicles favor the diagnosis of LEP. In contrast, the presence of adipocyte rimming by atypical lymphocytes is more suggestive of subcutaneous panniculitis-like T-cell lymphoma. In addition, both entities show similar immunophenotypic features, including potential loss of CD7 expression.

40. C

Primary cutaneous CD4-positive small/medium T-cell lymphoproliferative disorder commonly presents as a solitary nodule in the head and neck region. Microscopic examination typically reveals a dense or nodular dermal infiltrate with minimal to no epidermotropism. The infiltrate is composed of small to medium-sized pleomorphic lymphocytes admixed with occasional large cells. The infiltrate may contain an extensive inflammatory infiltrate composed of small B-lymphocytes, plasma cells, histiocytes and eosinophils. The neoplastic cells are CD3+, CD4+, CD8-, CD30-, EBV- and are negative for cytotoxic markers. They also show expression of markers associated with follicular helper T-cells such as PD-1, BCL-6 and CXCL-13. Patients are frequently asymptomatic and the disease shows an indolent clinical course.

41. D

Primary cutaneous CD8-positive aggressive epidermotropic cytotoxic T-cell lymphoma is an extremely rare primary cutaneous T-cell lymphoma characterized by marked epidermotropism and an aggressive clinical course. The disease is most common in adults and can present as either localized or widespread patches, plaques, papules and/or tumors with or without ulceration. Unlike mycosis fungoides, the disease is not initially limited to sun-protected sites and does not show a prolonged clinical course with slow progression of the lesions. In fact, there may be widespread dissemination at diagnosis (with sparing of the lymph nodes), and the disease has an aggressive clinical course with poor overall survival.

Microscopic examination of the lesions shows a dense, intraepidermal (pagetoid) infiltrate composed of small to intermediate-sized atypical lymphocytes admixed with variable amounts of large pleomorphic lymphocytes. Acanthosis, hyperkeratosis, dyskeratotic keratinocytes, epidermal ulceration and blister formation may also be present. The neoplastic cells may also localize to adnexal structures and show angioinvasion. The neoplastic cells are CD3+, CD4-, CD8+ with variable loss of CD2, CD5 and CD7. They are negative for CD30, CD56 and EBV-encoded RNA and have a TCR-αβ phenotype.

42. C

Lymphomatoid papulosis is chronic skin disorder most commonly seen in adult patients that is characterized by the presence of numerous cutaneous lesions in various stages of development (papules, nodules) that predominantly affect the trunk and extremities. The histologic appearance of the lesions is highly variable, and is partly dependent on the age of the lesion at the time of biopsy. The morphologic and immunophenotypic features of the lesions overlap with several types of cutaneous lymphoma. Diagnosis is aided by the tendency of the lesions to show spontaneous regression within weeks to months, leaving behind only hypopigmented or hyperpigmented scars. The disease is considered to be benign, but it may last from months to decades. Lymphomatous polyposis is a rare type of B-cell lymphoma, most frequently mantle cell lymphoma, characterized by the formation of numerous polyps along the gastrointestinal tract.

43. C

Lymphomatoid papulosis has three recognized histologic subtypes that show morphologic and immunophenotypic overlap with several types of cutaneous lymphoma.

Type A lesions are the most common and show a wedge-shaped dermal and perivascular infiltrate composed of large atypical lymphocytes with Hodgkin/Reed Sternberg-like morphology surrounded by an inflammatory infiltrate composed of neutrophils, small lymphocytes, histiocytes and eosinophils (mimicking classical Hodgkin lymphoma). The large atypical lymphocytes are frequently CD3+, CD4+, CD8- and CD30+.

Type B lesions are the least common and show an epidermotropic infiltrate composed of atypical lymphocytes with cerebriform morphology (mimicking mycosis fungoides). The atypical cells are frequently CD3+, CD4+, CD8- and may also express CD30.

Type C lesions show sheets of large atypical lymphocytes in the dermis with anaplastic,

horseshoe-shaped nuclei (mimicking primary cutaneous anaplastic large cell lymphoma). The neoplastic cells are CD3+, CD4+, CD8- and show strong, uniform expression of CD30 in the majority (>75%) of neoplastic cells. The neoplastic cells are negative for ALK-1, which helps to distinguish it from secondary cutaneous involvement by anaplastic large cell lymphoma, ALK-positive.

Of note, a Type D variant of lymphomatoid papulosis has been described, which shows histologic features similar to primary aggressive epidermotropic CD8+ cytotoxic T-cell lymphoma.

44. B

Primary cutaneous anaplastic large cell lymphoma may present as solitary or localized papules, nodules or tumors, often with ulceration. By definition, the disease is localized to the skin at diagnosis. Morphologic examination shows a dermal infiltrate composed of sheets of large atypical lymphocytes with anaplastic, horseshoe-shaped nuclei (referred to as hallmark cells), dispersed chromatin and prominent nucleoli.

The neoplastic cells are frequently CD3+, CD4+, CD8- and show strong uniform expression of CD30 by the majority (>75%) of cells. They also express cytotoxic markers such as granzyme B, perforin and TIA-1. They are negative for expression of ALK and lack the characteristic translocation of the *ALK* gene seen in systemic anaplastic large cell lymphoma. In addition, primary cutaneous disease is associated with an older age at diagnosis (>30 years of age) compared to systemic disease.

45. D

Extranodal NK/T-cell lymphoma is a rare, highly aggressive tumor that is strongly associated with Epstein-Barr virus (EBV) and is composed of cells with an NK-cell immunophenotype or in some cases, a cytotoxic T-cell immunophenotype. The tumor most commonly presents as an ulcerative nodule or mass in the nasal cavity, nasopharynx or upper aerodigestive tract (referred to as nasal type lesions) and may cause extensive invasion and destruction of adjacent soft tissue and bone (lethal midline granuloma). Extranasal disease is most frequently found in the skin, which shows a characteristic subcutaneous localization. Other areas such as the gastrointestinal tract, testes, lung and eye may be involved. By definition, primary lymph node localization is not seen, but regional lymph nodes may become involved as the disease progresses. The bone marrow and peripheral blood are *not* frequently involved at diagnosis.

46. C

Extranodal NK/T-cell lymphoma most frequently occurs in adults (median, 40–50 years of age) and is commonly found in patients of Asian, Mexican and South American descent. It is considered the most common type of primary nasal lymphoma, especially in Asian patients. It is highly associated with Epstein-Barr virus (EBV).

47. A

The neoplastic infiltrate of extranodal NK/T-cell lymphoma may contain a variable amount of small cells, intermediate-sized cells and large cells. The nuclei of the cells are usually irregular and may be folded, angulated or even anaplastic. Chromatin is variably dispersed and nucleoli may or may not be present. In addition, variable amounts of acute and chronic inflammation may be present in the background. The tumors show extensive ulceration and necrosis. A characteristic finding is the tendency of the neoplastic cells to surround and invade blood vessels (referred to as angiocentricity and angioinvasion) and cause destruction of the vessel wall (referred to as angiodestruction).

48. C

Extranodal NK/T-cell lymphoma shows an immunophenotype that is similar to NK-cells and is frequently CD2+, surface CD3-, cytoplasmic CD3+ and CD56+. The neoplastic cells also express cytotoxic molecules such as TIA-1, granzyme B and perforin. In-situ hybridization for EBV-encoded RNA (EBER) is positive.

49. D

Aggressive NK-cell leukemia is an extremely rare disorder that results from the proliferation of neoplastic NK-cells in the peripheral blood, bone marrow, and spleen. Cutaneous involvement is uncommon. It is most commonly seen in young adults (median, 30–40 years of age) of Asian descent.

The disease shows an aggressive clinical course; patients frequently present with "B symptoms", hepatosplenomegaly, fever and cytopenias, which may be accompanied by disseminated intravascular

coagulation (DIC) and hemophagocytic syndrome (HPS).

The neoplastic cells in the peripheral blood may resemble the normal large granular lymphocytes (LGLs) seen in reactive conditions or may show variable amounts of nuclear pleomorphism, dispersion of chromatin and prominent nucleoli. However, the presence of ample basophilic cytoplasm with prominent azurophilic granules is a useful diagnostic clue. Correct classification of these cells as either cytotoxic T-cells or NK-cells requires immunophenotypic analysis, and possibly molecular genetic analysis of the *TCR* gene to demonstrate a germline configuration consistent with NK-cell lineage.

The disease is almost universally associated with the presence of Epstein-Barr virus (EBV). Detection of EBV allows for differentiation with chronic lymphoproliferative disorders of NK-cells, which shows an indolent clinical course and is EBV-negative.

50. B

The clinical presentation of angioimmunoblastic T-cell lymphoma includes several characteristic findings that overlap with infectious/inflammatory and autoimmune disease. This unique presentation led to the initial classification of this disease as an abnormal immune reaction with increased risk of development of lymphoma. Most patients present with prominent systemic symptoms such as fever and weight loss. Other frequently encountered symptoms includes pruritic rash, edema, ascites, polyclonal hypergammaglobulinemia, cold agglutinins, cyroglobulins, Coombs-positive hemolytic anemia, arthritis, positive Rheumatoid factors, antismooth muscle antibodies and antinuclear antibodies.

51. D

Patients with angioimmunoblastic T-cell lymphoma frequently present with widespread, advanced stage disease at diagnosis. Generalized lymphadenopathy, hepatosplenomegaly, cutaneous involvement and bone marrow involvement are common.

In addition, the neoplasm appears to induce a secondary immunodeficiency which may lead to infectious disease complications and secondary neoplasms. Angioimmunoblastic T-cell lymphoma is almost always associated with the Epstein-Barr virus (EBV); however, the virus is not present in the neoplastic T-cells; instead the background B-cells, particularly immunoblasts, are infected with EBV.

The presence of disease-associated immunodeficiency as well as immunodeficiency secondary to chemotherapy may allow for progression to EBV-positive B-cell lymphoma, most frequently in the form of diffuse large B-cell lymphoma.

52. A

Angioimmunoblastic T-cell lymphoma shows a characteristic paracortical and interfollicular pattern of infiltration, which frequently extends past the lymph node capsule into the perinodal adipose tissue while simultaneously sparing the paracortical sinuses (so-called skip or jump pattern).

The infiltrate is often polymorphous and consists of small to intermediate-sized lymphocytes with round to irregular nuclei and abundant clear cytoplasm with prominent cell membranes. The morphology of the neoplastic cells is also quite variable. The cells may range from large and anaplastic to small with virtually no atypia. The infiltrate is admixed with, and may be obscured by, a prominent inflammatory infiltrate composed of eosinophils, plasma cells and histiocytes. The presence of variable amounts of B-cells with immunoblastic or Hodgkin/Reed-Sternberg-like morphology may also be seen.

A key morphologic finding is the presence of numerous expanded and "arborizing" high endothelial venules as well as the presence of expanded follicular dendritic cell meshworks in the paracortical, interfollicular and perinodal tissue (i.e. aberrant localization outside of follicles). Residual follicles may be present, and their appearance helps to define the three recognized "patterns" of angioimmunoblastic T-cell lymphoma.

53. B

Angioimmunoblastic T-cell lymphoma has three recognized architectural patterns (Patterns I, II and III) characterized by an increasing amount of lymph-node architectural effacement and characteristic morphology of background residual follicles. These patterns appear to represent consecutive morphologic stages of disease.

Pattern I, the earliest and less frequently encountered pattern, shows preservation of lymph node architecture with mild paracortical expansion and hyperplastic follicles without mantle zones.

Pattern II shows effacement of lymph-node architecture with paracortical expansion and occasional small, atretic follicles with "burned-out" germinal centers reminiscent of those seen in Castleman's Disease.

Pattern III, which is the most frequently encountered pattern, shows near-complete effacement of the lymph node architecture and near-complete absence of residual follicles.

54. A

The neoplastic cells of angioimmunoblastic T-cell lymphoma show pan T-cell antigen expression (CD2, CD3, CD5 and CD7) and are positive for CD4 and negative for CD8. The neoplastic cells have a follicular helper T-cell immunophenotype, which is a useful diagnostic tool.

Follicular helper T-cells are required for germinal center formation, maturation and development of germinal center cells and formation of plasma cells and memory cells. This T-cell subset is characterized by the expression of numerous markers including PD-1, BCL-6 and CXCL-13. Although CD10 is not a specific marker for follicular helper T-cells, its expression in the neoplastic cell infiltrate is an extremely useful tool for diagnosis.

In addition, antibodies against CD21, CD23 and CD35 are useful for visualizing the expanded follicular dendritic cell meshworks that characterize this disease. The presence of variable amounts of B-cells infected with EBV is another characteristic feature, which can be visualized by in situ hybridization studies for EBV-encoded RNA (EBER). The neoplastic T-cells are negative for EBV.

55. D

Anaplastic large cell lymphoma, ALK-positive, is characterized by the presence of large lymphoid cells with abundant eosinophilic cytoplasm, anaplastic nuclei resembling a horseshoe or kidney and a prominent eosinophilic region near the nucleus (referred to as "hallmark cells").

56. C

By definition, all cases of ALK-positive anaplastic large cell lymphoma show strong, uniform staining for CD30 (membranous and Golgi pattern) in virtually all of the neoplastic cells. This helps to differentiate from cases of CD30-positive peripheral T-cell lymphoma, in which CD30 expression is often weak and heterogeneous.

Although considered a T-cell neoplasm, anaplastic large cell lymphoma may show extensive loss of pan T-cell antigens. CD3, CD5, and CD7 are frequently absent; CD2 and CD4 are the most frequently detected antigens. Some cases have a "null-cell" phenotype characterized by a complete lack of pan T-cell antigen expression. Nevertheless the vast majority (90%) of cases of anaplastic large cell lymphoma will show clonal rearrangement of the *TCR* gene, regardless of T-cell antigen expression. Finally, expression of cytotoxic T-cell antigens such as TIA-1, granzyme B and perforin is seen in most cases.

57. A

The morphologic features of anaplastic large cell lymphoma, ALK-negative, can be heterogeneous but the presence of "hallmark cells" is found in all cases. The presence of a sinusoidal growth pattern in lymph nodes is another typical morphologic finding. The immunophenotype of ALK-negative cases is similar to ALK-positive cases in that virtually all (>75%) neoplastic cells show strong uniform expression of CD30 and frequent loss of pan T-cell antigen expression. The majority of cases are also positive for EMA and cytotoxic markers such as TIA-1, perforin and granzyme B.

ALK-negative cases show a worse prognosis than ALK-positive cases and present at a later median age. ALK-positive cases are more frequently seen in the first three decades of life while ALK-negative cases are more frequently found in patients in the 4th–7th decade of life.

58. A

The majority of cases of ALK-positive anaplastic large cell lymphoma are associated with t(2;5) (p23;q35), which juxtaposes the *ALK* gene on chromosome 2;p23 with the *NPM* gene on chromosome 5q35. The *ALK* gene codes for ALK (anaplastic lymphoma kinase), which is a tyrosine kinase receptor. The *NPM* gene codes for nucleophosmin, a chaperone protein which, in addition to many other functions, assists in the shuttling of other proteins into the nucleus.

The result of the translocation is an NPM-ALK fusion protein that forms homodimers with wild-type NPM protein. The wild-type NPM allows the fusion protein to enter the nucleus and also results in the activation of the tyrosine kinase domain of *ALK*. The end result is activation and upregulation of the ALK protein, resulting in oncogenesis.

At least 11 variant translocations have been identified, but all place the *ALK* gene under the influence of promoter sequences for constitutively activated genes; as such, all result in the upregulation of ALK.

Interestingly, the type of translocation affects the staining pattern seen with immunohistochemistry. The classic t(2;5) results in staining in the nucleus, nucleolus and cytoplasm, while other translocations result in different staining patterns. Nevertheless, the type of translocation does not appear to affect the clinicopathologic features of the disease.

59. B

The majority of patients with anaplastic large cell lymphoma, ALK-positive, will present with advanced stage disease. Nevertheless, the overall prognosis is good with five-year survival rates of 70–80%. Relapse occurs in approximately 30% of cases, but relapsed disease remains sensitive to chemotherapy.

60. C

Breast implant-associated anaplastic large cell lymphoma is a rare disease which most often presents as a large effusion or seroma surrounded by a thickened capsule adjacent to the underlying implant. A subset of patients will also develop a discreet mass. Histologic review often shows extensive fibrinoid necrosis and sclerosis. The neoplastic cells are large, epithelioid, with abundant eosinophilic cytoplasm and irregular to anaplastic nuclei. "Hallmark cells" with horseshoe-shaped nuclei are occasionally seen. The neoplastic cells show strong uniform expression of CD30 and are almost always negative for ALK.

61. D

Breast implant-associated anaplastic large cell lymphoma has an overall indolent clinical course. Patients who present with an effusion and no mass have an excellent prognosis after capsulectomy and removal of the breast implant. However, patients who also have a distinct mass appear to have a more aggressive clinical course and may require chemotherapy and/or radiation in addition to capsulectomy and implant removal.

62. C

Peripheral T-cell lymphoma, not otherwise specified (PTCL-NOS), is the preferred diagnosis for a mature T-cell neoplasm that does not meet criteria to be classified under any of the other World Health Organization–defined subtypes of mature T-cell lymphoma. As such, other subtypes of T-cell lymphoma must be excluded before diagnosis.

In order to keep these defined subtypes "pure," cases that display some of the characteristics of a World Health Organization–defined subtype but do not fulfil all the criteria for classification should still be classified as PTCL-NOS. It is recognized that the term PTCL-NOS likely encompasses several diseases and that further research will discover additional subtypes.

63. B

Due to the broad definition of peripheral T-cell lymphoma, not otherwise specified (PTCL-NOS), these tumors display a wide spectrum of morphologic and immunophenotypic findings. The neoplastic cells may range from small with minimal atypia to large with anaplastic nuclei. Cells with Hodgkin/Reed-Sternberg-like morphology may also be seen. An inflammatory background composed of eosinophils, histiocytes and plasma cells (imparting a "pink" appearance to hematoxylin and eosin-stained sections) is a frequent finding and useful diagnostic clue. Proliferation of high endothelial venules may also be seen, but in such cases, the presence of angioimmunoblastic T-cell lymphoma should be excluded. As mentioned, some cases of PTCL-NOS may display characteristics of other defined T-cell lymphoma subtypes. Expression of CD30, for example, would raise the possibility of anaplastic large cell lymphoma. However, anaplastic large cell lymphoma is defined as having strong, uniform expression of CD30. Therefore, cases that show only weak, heterogeneous of CD30, are better classified as PTCL-NOS.

64. D

Flow cytometry is a useful tool for detecting aberrant T-cell populations. Detection of altered expression (usually diminished expression or complete loss) of pan T-cell antigens such as CD2, CD3, CD5 and CD7 is suggestive of a T-cell neoplasm. CD5 and CD7 are the most frequently lost antigens in peripheral T-cell lymphoma, not otherwise specified. The detection of antigens not normally present on T-cells such as CD10, CD16, CD30 and so on is another useful diagnostic tool. HLA-DR expression can be seen on normal activated T-cells, and its presence alone is not sufficient to render a diagnosis of malignancy.

Hemostasis and Coagulopathy

Coagulation Disorders

Laboratory Analysis of Bleeding Disorders and Fibrinolysis: Questions 1–37

1. In light transmission platelet aggregometry, platelet function is tested by measuring the degree of platelet aggregation in response to platelet agonists. Which of the following are strong platelet agonists?
   A. ADP, thrombin, collagen
   B. ATP, thrombin, collagen
   C. Collagen, thrombin, thromboxane 2
   D. Epinephrine, collagen, ATP
   E. ADP, epinephrine, thrombin

2. In light transmission platelet aggregometry, what does the primary wave of aggregation represent after addition of the agonist ADP?
   A. Activation of the glycoprotein IIb/IIIa
   B. Platelet degranulation with recruitment of additional platelet aggregates
   C. Rearrangement of the platelet membrane phospholipid
   D. Binding of phospholipid-dependent coagulation complexes

3. Which platelet agonists show a biphasic pattern in light transmission platelet aggregometry?
   A. ATP and ADP
   B. ADP and epinephrine
   C. ATP and collagen
   D. ADP and thrombin

4. Which pattern of platelet aggregation would be seen in Von Willebrand's disease?

	ADP, primary	ADP, secondary	Arachidonic Acid	Epinephrine	Collagen	Ristocetin
A	decreased	decreased	decreased	decreased	decreased	N
B	increased	increased	increased	increased	increased	N
C	N	N	decreased	decreased	decreased	decreased
D	N	N	decreased	N	N	N
E	N	N	N	N	N	decreased

5. Which pattern of platelet aggregation would be seen in Scott syndrome?

	ADP, primary	ADP, secondary	Arachidonic Acid	Epinephrine	Collagen	Ristocetin
A	decreased	decreased	decreased	decreased	decreased	decreased
B	N	N	N	N	N	N
C	increased	increased	increased	increased	increased	increased
D	increased	increased	increased	decreased	decreased	decreased
E	decreased	decreased	decreased	increased	increased	increased

6. Which pattern of platelet aggregation would be seen in Glanzmann thrombasthenia or afibrinogenemia?

	ADP, primary	ADP, secondary	Arachidonic Acid	Epinephrine	Collagen	Ristocetin
A	absent	absent	absent	N	absent	absent
B	absent	absent	absent	absent	N	absent
C	absent	absent	absent	absent	absent	N
D	absent	absent	N	absent	absent	absent
E	N	N	absent	absent	absent	absent

7. Which pattern of platelet aggregation is seen in dense granule platelet storage pool disorders?

	ADP, primary	ADP, secondary	Arachidonic Acid	Epinephrine	Collagen	Ristocetin
A	N	decreased	N	N or decreased	N or decreased	N
B	N or decreased	N or decreased	N	N	N	N
C	N	N or decreased	decreased	decreased	decreased	N
D	decreased	N or decreased	N	N	N	N
E	N	N	decreased	N	decreased	N

8. Which of the following patterns would be seen in Bernard-Soulier syndrome?

	ADP, primary	ADP, secondary	Arachidonic Acid	Epinephrine	Collagen	Ristocetin
A	N	N	N	N	decreased or absent	N
B	N	N	N	decreased or absent	N	N
C	N	N	N	N	N	decreased or absent
D	N	N	decreased or absent	N	N	N
E	N	decreased or absent	N	N	N	N

9. Which pattern would be seen in a patient taking aspirin?

	ADP, primary	ADP, secondary	Arachidonic Acid	Epinephrine	Collagen	Ristocetin
A	decreased	decreased	N	decreased	N	N
B	N	N	absent	decreased	Decreased or absent	N
C	N	decreased	absent	decreased	Decreased or absent	N
D	decreased	N	absent	decreased	Decreased or absent	N
E	decreased	decreased	absent	decreased	decreased	N

10. The thromboelastogram (TEG) is a viscoelastic test that characterizes the strength and formation of a clot over time. A blood sample is introduced into the oscillating cup of the TEG machine, and a torsion wire connected to a detector is placed into the blood. As the cup rotates and coagulation occurs, the pin moves with the clot, and the kinetics of clot formation is graphically displayed by the computer. Several parameters are measured: R (reaction time), k (k time), α angle, MA (maximum amplitude), LY30 (lysis at 30 min.), CI (coagulation index). Which of the following is a true statement concerning these parameters?

    A. A clotting factor deficiency would cause a shortening of the R time

    B. During hyperfibrinolysis, the LY30 would decrease

    C. Thrombocytopenia would result in an elevated MA

    D. During hyperfibrinolysis, the k and α angle would decrease

11. What is the cause of this abnormal TEG?

R min (4–8)	K min (1–4)	Angle Deg (47–74)	MA mm (55–73)	CI (-3-3)	LY30 % (0–8)
7.8	4.5	37.5	57	-4.8	0

A. Hypofibrinogenemia

B. DIC

C. Clotting factor deficiency

D. Thrombocytopenia

12. A 64-year-old patient undergoes a laparotomy for pneumoperitoneum. The operation occurs uneventfully and adequate hemostasis is achieved. Three hours later the patient begins to bleed from the abdominal wound. A TEG is performed and the results are shown. What is the cause of the bleeding?

R min (4–8)	K min (1–4)	Angle Deg (47–74)	MA mm (55–73)	CI (-3-3)	LY30 % (0–8)
5.2	1.5	69	60	2	0.4

A. Residual heparin

B. Lupus anticoagulant

C. Surgical bleeding

D. DIC

13. Which TEG tracing pattern is consistent with primary (hyper)fibrinolysis?

	R min (4–8)	K min (1–4)	Angle Deg (47–74)	MA mm (55–73)	CI (-3-3)	LY30 % (0–8)
A	3.7	1.2	74.9	48	0.7	45
B	3.4	1	76	80	3.5	40
C	3.4	1	76	80	0.6	42
D	3.2	1.2	75	49	3.5	30

14. Which of the following is true of the euglobulin clot lysis time (ECLT)?

    A. An ECLT of < 30 minutes demonstrates hypofibrinolysis

    B. The euglobulin fraction of plasma contains fibrinogen, plasminogen activators and plasminogen

    C. After precipitating plasma at low pH, the remaining supernatant is clotted with thrombin and the time to clot lysis is measured

    D. An ECLT between 60 and 120 minutes demonstrates hypofibrinoloysis

15. Which of the following could be used to diagnose Factor XIII deficiency?

    A. Thromboelastogram

    B. Platelet aggregation studies

C. Russell viper venom test

D. Urea clot lysis

E. Ristocetin cofactor assay

16. Which of the following would cause a false positive result in the urea clot lysis test?

A. A transfusion of 1 unit of FFP

B. Antiplasmin deficiency

C. Aminocaproic acid therapy

D. Heterozygous status for Factor XIII deficiency

17. A 47-year-old patient with congestive heart failure undergoes coagulation testing prior to cardiac surgery. The following values are obtained:

PT – 12.2 [10.5–14.0]

PTT – 45.0 [22.0–34.0]

Thrombin time – 22s [13–15s]

Reptilase time – 14s [13–15s]

The patient most likely has:

A. An acquired Factor VIII inhibitor

B. Taken unfractionated heparin

C. Taken fish oil supplementation

D. Dysfibrinogenemia

18. Which of the following statements is true concerning the reptilase time and/or thrombin time?

A. Disseminated intravascular coagulation results in a decrease in both the reptilase time and thrombin time

B. Reptilase cleaves fibrinogen releasing fibrinopeptide A and fibrinopeptide B

C. Reptilase is isolated from Bothrops atrox

D. Thrombin time cleaves fibrinogen releasing fibrinopeptide A

19. Increased thrombin and reptilase times may be seen in:

A. A neonate

B. A patient on warfarin

C. A patient on direct thrombin inhibitors

D. A patient with a heparin-like anticoagulant

20. A 45-year-old man with Crohn's disease undergoes a third operation for complications arising from an intestinal obstruction. The many adhesions from previous surgeries results in prolonged bleeding and oozing from the surgical site. Bovine thrombin is applied topically, and hemostasis is eventually attained. The patient has no issues postoperatively; however, on day 9 there is elevation of the PT to 45s (11–14s) and PTT to 150s (25–35s) with bleeding at the surgical site. Mixing studies do not correct. A peripheral blood smear is normal. What is the cause of the coagulopathy?

A. Factor inhibitor

B. Disseminated intravascular coagulation

C. Acute liver failure

D. Acquired Von Willebrand disease

E. Vitamin K deficiency

21. Which of the following laboratory findings best represents type IIb Von Willebrand disease?

	VWF:Ag	VWF:RCo	FVIII:C	VWF:RCo/ VWF:Ag ratio	Multimers	RIPA
A	dec	dec	dec or normal	> 0.6	dec HMW multimers	inc
B	dec	dec	dec or normal	> 0.6	dec HMW multimers	dec
C	dec	dec	dec or normal	< 0.6	dec HMW multimers	dec
D	dec	dec	dec or normal	< 0.6	dec HMW multimers	inc

22. Which set of laboratory values would most likely be seen in type IIa Von Willebrand disease?

	VWF:Ag	VWF:RCo	FVIII:C	VWF:RCo/ VWF:Ag ratio	Multimers	RIPA
A	dec	dec	dec or normal	< 0.6	dec HMW multimers	dec or normal
B	dec	dec	dec or normal	< 0.6	dec HMW multimers	inc or normal
C	dec	dec	dec or normal	< 0.6	dec HMW multimers	inc
D	dec	dec	dec or normal	< 0.6	dec LMW multimers	dec or normal

23. Which set of laboratory values would most likely be seen in type IIM Von Willebrand disease?

	VWF:Ag	VWF:RCo	FVIII:C	VWF:RCo/ VWF:Ag ratio	Multimers	RIPA
A	normal	dec	dec or normal	> 0.6	Low LMW multimers	reduced
B	normal or decreased	dec	dec or normal	< 0.6	Normal	reduced
C	normal	dec	dec or normal	< 0.6	Low HMW multimers	reduced
D	dec	normal	dec or normal	< 0.6	Low HMW multimers	reduced

24. Which set of laboratory values would most likely be seen in type III Von Willebrand disease?

	VWF:Ag	VWF:RCo	FVIII:C	VWF:RCo/ VWF:Ag ratio	Multimers	RIPA
A	absent	absent	decreased	< 0.6	dec HMW multimers	absent
B	absent	absent	decreased	> 0.6	low HMW multimers	absent
C	absent	absent	decreased	< 0.6	absent	absent
D	absent	absent	decreased	< 0.6	Low HMW multimers	absent

25. Which of the following values would be expected to be seen in type I VWD?
    A. Normal VWF:RCo
    B. Increased VWF:Ag
    C. Increased Factor VIII:C
    D. VWF:RCo/VWF:Ag ratio > 0.6
    E. Decreased intermediate molecular weight multimers

26. A 46-year-old patient with uterine cancer is hospitalized for surgery. A central line is placed; however, oozing occurs at the site of placement.

A coagulopathy workup is performed with the following results:

Platelet – 275 × 10³/L

PT – 13s (11–14s)

PTT – 34s (25–35s)

Fibrinogen – 150 mg/dL (150–400 mg/dL)

FDP – >20 ug/mL (<10 ug/mL)

D-dimer – >250 ng/mL (< or = 250 ng/mL)

Which of the following is the likely diagnosis?

A. Chronic DIC

B. Afibrinogenemia

C. Dysfibrinogenemia

D. Surgical bleeding

27. A 5-year-old male develops spontaneous epistaxis while playing basketball. Coagulation workup is initiated. The following laboratory values are obtained:

Platelet – 325 × 10³/L

PT – 13s (11–14s)

PTT – 70s (25–35s)

Which of the following is the next best test?

A. Factor activity for Factor VII

B. Mixing study

C. Thromboelastography (TEG)

D. Platelet aggregation study

E. Fibrinogen

28. A hematology researcher does extensive coagulation testing on the the patient described in question #27 including TEG, platelet aggregation studies, fibrinogen, mixing studies and thrombin time. A mixing study shows evidence of correction of the PTT into reference range. Which is the most likely coagulopathy affecting the patient in question #27?

A. Factor VIII inhibitor

B. Lupus anticoagulant

C. Factor V inhibitor

D. Factor XI deficiency

29. A 7-year-old child presents to the E.R. with several deep bruises in his arms and legs after playing football. In addition, he reports having nosebleeds once a month. The following laboratory values are obtained:

Platelet – 200 × 10³/L

PT – 14s (11–14s)

PTT – 65s (25–35s)

Mixing studies show correction of the PTT into reference range.

This patient's diagnosis is:

A. Child abuse

B. Von Willebrand disease

C. Hemophilia B

D. Ehlers-Danlos syndrome

30. A new platelet function analyser (PFA-100) is purchased by a Laboratory Medicine Department. The PFA-100 consists of test cartridges with membranes coated with collagen and adenosine diphosphate (ADP) or collagen and epinephrine (EPI). As citrated whole blood is aspirated through an aperture in the membrane, the device measures the amount of time it takes for the aperture to close. The following results are obtained on a sample specimen:

Collagen-EPI: 235s (78–199s)

Collagen-ADP: 78s (55–137s)

What is the diagnosis:

A. Von Willebrand disease

B. Aspirin use

C. Gray platelet syndrome

D. Liver disease

31. Which test or method might allow a lab clinician to differentiate between type 2B VWD and pseudo-platelet type VWD?

A. Ristocetin-induced agglutination of washed patient platelets mixed with normal plasma

B. VWF multimer analysis

C. Ristocetin-induced platelet aggregation

D. Thrombocytopenia

32. What are the components of the activated partial thromboplastin time (aPTT)?

A. Tissue factor, phospholipid, calcium

B. Prothrombin, phospholipid, calcium

C. Thrombin, phospholipid, calcium

D. Silica, phospholipid, calcium

33. What condition results in a shortened aPTT?

A. Lupus anticoagulant

B. Factor XI inhibitor

C. Elevated Factor VIII levels

D. High hematocrit levels

34. What is the formula for the international normalized ratio?

A. $(PT\ measured/PT\ mean)^{ISI}$

B. $(PTmeasured-PTmean/PTmean)^{ISI}$

C. $(PTmean/PTmeasured)^{ISI}$

D. $(PTmean-PTmeasured/PTmeasured)^{ISI}$

35. In which situation is the activated clotting time (ACT) used?

A. To monitor warfarin therapy

B. To monitor low molecular weight heparin

C. To monitor high doses of unfractionated heparin

D. To monitor direct Factor Xa inhibitors

36. For which of the following conditions is the anti-Factor Xa assay most useful?
    A. Diagnosing a Factor X inhibitor
    B. Monitoring low molecular weight heparin therapy
    C. Indirectly measuring PTT
    D. Diagnosing a Factor X deficiency

37. Which of the following is true of the anti-Factor Xa assay?
    A. The therapeutic range of UFH for treatment of DVT is 1–2 U/mL.
    B. Must be collected 30 minutes after injection of LMWH
    C. Is affected by abnormal factor levels
    D. Usually a chromogenic assay

Laboratory Analysis of Thrombotic Disorders: Questions 38–47

38. How is the ratio derived from the activated protein C (APC) resistance assay expressed?
    A. (PT + APC) / aPTT
    B. (PTT + APC) / PT
    C. (PT + APC) / PT
    D. (aPTT + APC) /aPTT

39. An APC resistance assay is performed on a patient who developed a deep venous thrombosis after surgery despite being on heparin. The APC resistance ratio is 2.2. What can be said about Factor V Leiden mutation in this patient?
    A. The patient does not have a Factor V Leiden mutation
    B. The patient is homozygous for Factor V Leiden mutation
    C. The patient is heterozygous for Factor V Leiden mutation

40. Which of the following patterns represent platelet hypercoagulability on thromboelastography (TEG) tracing?

	R min (4–8)	K min (1–4)	Angle Deg (47–74)	MA mm (55–73)	CI (-3-3)
A	3.9	1.5	56	60	3.5
B	2.5	1.2	76	55	1.5
C	6.2	1.3	76	78.2	3.1
D	4	3	43	52	1.6

41. Which of the following patterns would be seen in antithrombin deficiency on thromboelastography (TEG) tracing?

	R min (4–8)	K min (1–4)	Angle Deg (47–74)	MA mm (55–73)	CI (-3-3)
A	9	2	65	74	3.6
B	3	5	60	70	3.5
C	1.5	1.3	75	65	3.8
D	2	2	70	70	3.6

42. What is the gold standard for diagnosis of heparin-induced thrombocytopenia?
    A. Ultrasound demonstration of thrombosis after heparin use
    B. Serotonin release assay
    C. Heparin/PF4 ELISA
    D. Heparin-induced platelet aggregation

43. Which of the following is true of anti-PF4-heparin enzyme immunoassays for the diagnosis of heparin induced thromboctyopenia (HIT)?
    A. Clinically evident HIT develops in a majority (60–80%) of heparin-treated patients who have anti-PF4-heparin antibodies detected by this immunoassay
    B. Anti-PF4-heparin antibodies are present only after the platelet count begins to decline
    C. Seroconversion after an initially negative test for anti-PF4-heparin antibodies almost always detect clinically relevant antibodies
    D. Anti-PF4-heparin enzyme immunoassays have high negative predictive values

44. Which of the following is true of the D-dimer test?
    A. D-dimer is the degradation product of fibrin crosslinked by Factor XII
    B. D-dimer is usually decreased in the setting of pregnancy, inflammation, malignancy and trauma
    C. Lipemia, elevated serum rheumatoid factor level, hyperbilirubinemia and hemolylsis may falsely increase the D-dimer level
    D. Deep venous thrombosis (DVT) cannot be ruled out in a patient who is clinically judged not to have DVT combined with a negative D-dimer test

45. Which of the following is an immunoassay used for the detection of antiphospholipid antibodies?
    A. Anti-β2-glycoprotein I IgG and IgM
    B. Kaolin clotting time (KCT)
    C. Dilute Russell viper venom test
    D. anticardiolipid IgG and IgM

46. Which of the following is a true statement?
    A. Anti-β2-GPI assays are the most sensitive for detecting antiphospholipid antibodies
    B. Anti-β2-GPI positivity is associated with an increased risk of myocardial infarction
    C. Anti-β2-GPI assays are the most specific for detecting antiphospholipid antibodies
    D. Presence of lupus anticoagulant is a major risk factor for arterial thrombotic events in young women

47. A 27-year-old woman with three previous miscarriages during the first trimester has a workup for antiphospholipid antibody syndrome. The PTT is prolonged and a mixing study fails to correct. The dilute Russell viper venom test shows a negative result. What is the next step in management?
    A. No further management. The patient has antiphospholipid antibody syndrome based on clinical criteria and prolonged PTT which fails to correct
    B. Perform an anti-β2-glycoprotein antibody test
    C. Perform factor activity for Factor VII
    D. Perform kaolin clotting time

Normal Physiology and Disorders of Primary Hemostasis: Questions 48–68

48. The dense granules of platelets contain many molecules. Which of the following is found in dense granules?
    A. Serotonin
    B. VEGF
    C. VWF
    D. PDGF
    E. Multimerin

49. Which platelet glycoprotein is the main binding receptor for fibrinogen?
    A. Gp Ia/IIa
    B. Gp VI
    C. Gp Ib-IX-V
    D. Gp IIb/IIIa

50. Where can Von Willebrand factor (VWF) be found in the body?
    A. Delta granules of platelets
    B. Weibel-Palade bodies
    C. Kupffer cells
    D. Merkel cells

51. What molecule(s) do(es) endothelial cells secrete that prevents platelet aggregation?
    A. Prostaglandin I2
    B. Nitric oxide
    C. A and B
    D. None of the above

52. People with which blood group have the lowest mean levels of VWF?
    A. O
    B. A
    C. B
    D. AB

53. Which of the following disorders may have a reduction in both alpha and delta granules?
    A. Quebec syndrome
    B. Gray platelet syndrome
    C. Sebastian anomaly
    D. Wiskott-Aldrich syndrome
    E. Heparin-induced thrombocytopenia

54. Which of the following disorders is NOT caused by a mutation in the MYH9 gene?
    A. Sebastian syndrome
    B. Fechtner's syndrome
    C. Paris-Trousseau syndrome
    D. May-Hegglin anomaly
    E. Epstein syndrome

55. What is the most common inherited bleeding disorder?
    A. Hemophilia A
    B. Hemophilia B
    C. Von Willebrand disease
    D. Factor XI deficiency

56. Which of the following is inherited in an autosomal dominant fashion?
    A. Type III Von Willebrand disease
    B. Type IIN (Normandy) VWD
    C. Pseudo/platelet-type VWD
    D. Type IIb VWD

57. Type IIN (Normandy) Von Willebrand disease is a qualitative disorder that results in:
    A. A mutation in the VWF domain that binds Factor VIII
    B. Enhanced ristocetin induced platelet aggregation
    C. A mutation in VWF that prevents binding to platelet GP1b
    D. A mutation that interferes with VWF assembly

58. A 25-year-old woman at 15 weeks' gestation was admitted to the hospital for vaginal bleeding. An ultrasound confirmed a fetal death secondary to placental abruption. She successfully underwent suction dilatation and curettage; however, she began to bleed heavily an hour after the procedure. She was given 2 units of RBCs and 1 unit of platelets, and the bleeding stopped. Eight days after admission, she had recurring vaginal bleeding. Her platelet count was 5×10^9 / L; peripheral blood showed only decreased platelets; and PT, PTT, fibrinogen and fibrin split products were all within normal range. What is the cause for her coagulopathy?
    A. Disseminated intravascular coagulation (DIC)
    B. Post-transfusion purpura (PTP)
    C. Hyperfibrinolysis
    D. Immune thrombocytopenic purpura (ITP)

59. A 34-year-old woman is referred to a hematologist for the evaluation of anemia. On physical examination, she exhibits multiple blanching lesions on her lips, fingers and nose. In addition, she reports a history of spontaneous epistaxis and a family history of the same disorder in multiple family members. A CBC, PT and PTT are ordered and show no abnormalities. What is the likely diagnosis?
    A. Osler-Weber-Rendu syndrome
    B. Scleroderma
    C. Kasabach-Merritt syndrome

D. Louis-Bar syndrome
E. Liver disease

60. A full-term baby at 5 days of age was referred to a pediatric surgeon for the management of a 7 × 6 cm violaceous swelling on the lateral chest wall. An ultrasound showed a heterogeneous mass with increased vascularity. Abnormal laboratory studies demonstrated a platelet count of 40,000 and an elevated D-dimer. Which of the following is the appropriate diagnosis?
    A. Infantile hemangioma with hyperfibrinolysis
    B. Hereditary hemorrhagic telangiectasia
    C. Kasabach-Merritt syndrome
    D. von Hippel Landau disease
    E. Cutis marmorata telangiectatica congenita

61. What is the most common cause of hemolytic uremic syndrome (HUS) in children?
    A. *Shigella dysenteriae*
    B. *Camypylobacter*
    C. *Streptococcus pneumoniae*
    D. *Escherichia coli*

62. A 40-year-old woman with fever and epigastric pain of four days' duration presents to the emergency room. Her hematocrit is 24%, platelet count is 15×10^3/L, LDH is 899 U/L and peripheral smear shows schistocytes. What is the cause of this disorder?
    A. Deficiency of Von Willebrand factor
    B. Deficiency of ADAMTS 13
    C. Hypertensive crisis
    D. Sepsis

63. Which of the following is true of hereditary hemorrhagic telangiectasia (HHT)?
    A. Adult HHT patients do not typically exhibit iron deficiency anemia
    B. Nosebleeds occur during the latest stages of disease
    C. HHT has an incidence of approximately 1 in 80,000
    D. HHT may be caused by mutations in endoglin and ALK-1

64. Which of the following is true regarding the pathophysiology of uremic platelet dysfunction?
    A. The degree of azotemia correlates with bleeding risk

B. Urea is the major platelet toxin causing uremic platelet dysfunction resulting in abnormal expression of platelet glycoproteins

C. Patients with familial azotemia demonstrate normal in vitro platelet function

D. Contributing factors to uremic platelet dysfunction include increased prostaglandin metabolism and increased platelet thromboxane A2 generation

65. The effects of cardiopulmonary bypass on platelets show:

A. Normal platelet reactivity in vitro

B. Normal platelet reactivity in response to an in vivo wound

C. Loss of the platelet surface GPIb-IX and GPIIb-IIIa complexes

D. Increased number of degranulating platelets

66. A family brought their 2-year-old son to a pediatrician for clinical management and counseling. On physical examination, it was found that the boy has narrow palpebral fissures, small low set ears, cleft palate, and his past medical history was notable for developmental delay and febrile seizures. Genetic testing show a 22q11.2 deletion. What other laboratory finding is often seen with this disorder?

A. Shortened PT

B. Prolonged PT

C. Thrombocytopenia

D. Afibrinogenemia

67. Which of the following clinical manifestations is seen in thrombocytopenia and qualitative platelet disorders?

A. Petechiae

B. Hemarthrosis

C. Deep hematomas

D. Delayed bleeding

68. Which of the following drugs blocks the P2Y12 platelet receptor that mediates ADP-induced platelet activation?

A. Abciximab

B. Eptifibatide

C. Dipyridamole

D. Ticlopidine

Normal Physiology and Disorders of Secondary Hemostasis: Questions 69–85

69. Which of the following is not a vitamin K dependent clotting factor?

A. Factor XII

B. Factor II

C. Factor VII

D. Factor X

E. Factor IX

70. Which factors are part of the intrinsic system of the coagulation cascade?

A. II, VII, IX, X

B. VII, TF

C. X, V, II, I

D. VIII, IX, XI, XII

E. II, V, VIII, X

71. Which coagulopathy is associated with amyloidosis?

A. Factor V inhibitor

B. Factor X deficiency

C. Factor VIII inhibitor

D. Factor V deficiency

E. Plasminogen activator inhibitor-1

72. Which factor has the shortest plasma half-life?

A. Factor IX

B. Factor XI

C. Factor VII

D. Factor I

E. Factor X

73. Which factor has the longest plasma half-life?

A. Factor IX

B. Factor XIII

C. Factor I

D. Factor VII

E. Factor II

74. Which of the following is a true statement about protein S?

A. Protein S tends to be lower in men than women

B. Oral contraceptive use increases the level of protein S in the body

C. Protein S is low at birth but increases to adult reference range by 12 months

D. Protein S decreases due to an acute thrombotic event

E. Warfarin and vitamin K deficiency have no effect on protein S

75. What is the mechanism of action of acquired protein S deficiency during acute phase reactions like injury or stress?

A. The body consumes great quantities of protein S during an acute phase reaction

B. Protein S is necessary for adequate hemostasis during an acute phase reaction

C. C4b binding protein (C4bBP) is elevated during an acute phase reaction and binds to protein S

D. Protein S functions as a cofactor to protein C during acute phase reactions and inactivates Factors Va and VIIIa

76. Which of the following would result in an increase in free protein S levels?

A. Familial C4b binding protein deficiency

B. Pregnancy

C. Disseminated intravascular coagulation

D. Liver failure

E. Nephrotic syndrome

77. A 29-year-old medical student has just completed a riveting rotation in Hematology and decides to check his own coagulation status in the chemistry lab. Incidentally, he finds an elevated PTT but normal PT. Prolonged incubation results in the shortening of the PTT. He has no history of excessive bleeding. Which of the following is the cause of the isolated increase in PTT?

A. DIC

B. Vitamin K deficiency

C. Prekallikrein deficiency

D. Hemophilia A

E. Heparin contamination of blood sample

78. The same medical student as in question #77 eventually becomes a hematology fellow and interviews a hospitalized patient who also has an isolated prolonged PTT. On further questioning, the patient, who was admitted for abdominal pain and vomiting, reports no history

of excessive bleeding in the past. Given this incidental finding in a patient without obvious coagulopathy, which of the following could be deficient in the patient?

A. High molecular weight kininogen

B. Low molecular weight kininogen

C. Factor VIII

D. Factor IX

E. Factor XI

79. Which of the following is true about Factor VII deficiency?

A. Factor VII deficiency is protective against thrombosis

B. Congenital Factor VII deficiency is an autosomal recessive disorder

C. Both PT and PTT are prolonged in Factor VII deficiency

D. Plasma is the treatment of choice for bleeding and surgery in Factor VII deficient patients

80. Which of the following conditions has the highest incidence of disseminated intravascular coagulation (DIC)?

A. Solid tumors

B. Aortic aneurysm

C. Advanced lung cancer

D. Sepsis/severe infection

81. Which of the following statements concerning disseminated intravascular coagulation is true?

A. Bacterial infection may induce coagulation directly via the induction of tissue factor expression on neutrophils

B. Antithrombin is continuously consumed during ongoing activation of coagulation

C. Fibrin-degradation products are decreased in DIC

D. Factor VIII is the central mediator of DIC in sepsis

82. Congenital dysfibrinogenemia:

A. Uncommonly causes thrombosis

B. Results in prolongation of the PT and PTT but not the thrombin time

C. Is inherited as an autosomal recessive trait

D. Is usually caused by a deletion in any of the three fibrinogen genes

83. The mode of inheritance for Hemophilia B is:
    A. Autosomal dominant
    B. Autosomal recessive
    C. X-linked dominant
    D. X-linked recessive
    E. Mitochondrial

84. Which of the following drugs enhances the capacity of antithrombin to inactivate thrombin and Factor Xa?
    A. Fondaparinux
    B. Heparin
    C. Lepirudin
    D. Apixaban

85. Which of the following is a direct Xa inhibitor?
    A. Apixaban
    B. Bivalirudin
    C. Low molecular weight heparin
    D. Dabigtran

Thrombotic Disorders: Questions 86–96

86. A 62-year-old multiparous woman with severe congestive heart failure undergoes cardiac surgery to implant a left ventricular assist device (LVAD) as a bridge to heart transplantation. She has moderate bleeding during the operation which requires one unit of RBCs, one dose of platelets and one FFP. Unfractionated heparin (UFH) prophylaxis is initiated immediately after surgery to prevent deep vein thrombosis. On the sixth postoperative day, the patient's platelet count falls from a baseline of $221 \times 10^9/$L to $104 \times 10^9/$L with no other abnormalities in the CBC. The physical exam is noncontributory. A peripheral blood smear demonstrates *no* schistocytes, giant platelets or satellitosis. A DIC panel shows increased D-dimer and normal fibrinogen, PT, PTT and INR.
    Which of the following is the most likely diagnosis?
    A. Splenomegaly
    B. Heparin-induced thrombocytopenia
    C. Post-transfusion purpura
    D. Disseminated intravascular coagulation
    E. Mechanical destruction by cardiopulmonary bypass circuit

87. Which of the following are risk factors for heparin-induced thrombocytopenia (HIT)? Choose all that apply:
    A. Orthopedic surgery
    B. Men
    C. Women
    D. Low molecular weight heparin
    E. Unfractionated heparin
    F. Long-term hemodialysis

88. Heparin-induced thrombocytopenia is caused by antibodies to multimolecular complexes of heparin and Platelet Factor-4 (PF4). Where is PF4 released from?
    A. Alpha granules of platelets
    B. Delta granules of platelets
    C. Endothelial cells
    D. Hepatocytes

89. What is a suitable alternative anticoagulant to heparin in a patient who develops heparin-induced thrombocytopenia (HIT)?
    A. Warfarin
    B. Phenprocoumon
    C. Abciximab
    D. Danaproid

90. A 52-year-old man was admitted to the hospital for his swollen and tender left leg after a long trip. A venogram showed a deep venous thrombosis and he was placed on heparin intravenously. A PT, PTT, platelet count and CBC were all normal. He was initiated on warfarin therapy and heparin was later discontinued. He was discharged after becoming therapeutic. He returned to the hospital the next day because of shortness of breath and pleuritic chest pain. A chest X-ray and findings of a ventilation-perfusion scan confirmed the presence of a pulmonary embolism. Additional laboratory studies for protein C, protein S, Factor V Leiden and antithrombin were normal. Which of the following is the patient's most likely diagnosis?
    A. Heparin-induced thrombocytopenia
    B. Dysfibrinogenemia
    C. Trousseau's syndrome
    D. Antithrombin deficiency
    E. Homocysteinemia

91. Activated protein C resistance due to Factor V Leiden is caused by which of the following?
    A. A point mutation in Factor V
    B. An autoantibody to activated protein C
    C. A deletion in protein C
    D. A point mutation in protein C
    E. Abnormal thrombin binding to Factor V

92. Which of the following thrombotic disorders is the most common inherited cause of venous thromboembolism?
    A. Protein S deficiency
    B. Protein C deficiency
    C. Prothrombin G20210A mutation
    D. Factor V Leiden
    E. Antithrombin deficiency

93. Which of the following disorders is inherited in an autosomal recessive fashion?
    A. Protein S deficiency
    B. Protein C deficiency
    C. Antithrombin deficiency
    D. Prothrombin mutation
    E. Homocysteinemia

94. Which of the following statements is true of the Prothrombin Gene G20210A mutation?
    A. The prevalence of the mutation is highest in Africa
    B. The mutation occurs in the 3' untranslated region of the prothrombin gene which substitutes an adenine for a guanine at position 20,210
    C. The presence of Factor V Leiden mutation in combination with the prothrombin gene mutation confers a twofold thrombotic risk above the risk of a single defect
    D. Plasma prothrombin concentrations can be used to screen for the prothrombin gene mutation

95. Antiphospholipid syndrome (APS) has which of the following characteristics?
    A. The majority of APS patients develop catastrophic antiphospholipid syndrome
    B. APS most commonly causes venous thrombosis in deep veins of the upper limbs

C. APS most commonly causes arterial thrombosis in cerebral arterial circulation
D. Diagnosis requires that only certain clinical criteria are met

96. Which of the following is true of hyperhomocysteinemia?
    A. There is an association between hyperhomocysteinemia and VTE and arterial thrombosis
    B. Homozygous deficiency of cystathionine-α-synthase results in homocystinuria
    C. Mutations in 5,10-methylene-tetrahydrofolate reductase (MTHFR) often lead to homocystinuria
    D. Homozygosity for the C677T mutation in MTHFR is a strong risk factor for arterial thrombosis

Disorders of Fibrinolysis: Questions 97–100

97. Which of the following enzymes is the primary inhibitor of tissue-type plasminogen activator (t-PA) and urokinase-type plasminogen activator (u-PA)?
    A. α2-antiplasmin
    B. TAFI
    C. PAI-1
    D. TFPI

98. Which is the best treatment option for the hemorrhagic tendency in primary fibrinolysis?
    A. Cryoprecipitate
    B. Fresh frozen plasma
    C. Argatroban
    D. Aminocaproic acid

99. Which of the following statements is true regarding acquired disorders of fibrinolysis?
    A. There is increased fibrinolytic activity in the endometrium of women with an intrauterine device (IUD) associated with menorrhagia
    B. A greater degree of hyperfibrinolysis in severe trauma patients confers a greater risk of survival
    C. Accelerated fibrinolysis during orthotopic liver transplantation (OLT) is associated with increased plasma t-PA, α2-antiplasmin and elevated fibrin-degradation products

D. Patients with amyloidosis and hyperfibrinolysis do not respond well to antifibrinolytic therapy

100. Which of the following statements is correct?

A. Type 1 plasminogen deficiency is associated with the development of ligneous conjunctivitis

B. Type 2 plasminogen deficiency is a quantitative disorder

C. Type 1 plasminogen deficiency is associated with a high risk of recurrent deep venous thromboembolism

D. The 36th College of American Pathologists Consensus Conference (2001) recommended including plasminogen activity in thrombophilia evaluations

Answers to Chapter 7

1. C	26. A	51. C	76. A
2. A	27. B	52. A	77. C
3. B	28. D	53. D	78. A
4. E	29. C	54. C	79. B
5. B	30. B	55. C	80. D
6. C	31. A	56. D	81. B
7. A	32. D	57. A	82. A
8. C	33. C	58. B	83. D
9. C	34. A	59. A	84. B
10. D	35. C	60. C	85. A
11. A	36. B	61. D	86. B
12. C	37. D	62. B	87. A,C, E
13. A	38. D	63. D	88. A
14. B	39. A	64. C	89. D
15. D	40. C	65. A	90. C
16. B	41. C	66. C	91. A
17. B	42. B	67. A	92. D
18. C	43. D	68. D	93. E
19. A	44. C	69. A	94. B
20. A	45. A	70. D	95. C
21. D	46. D	71. B	96. A
22. A	47. B	72. C	97. C
23. B	48. A	73. B	98. D
24. C	49. D	74. D	99. A
25. D	50. B	75. C	100. A

Answers to Chapter 7 (with Explanations)

1. **C**

   There are two types of platelet agonists, strong and weak. Strong agonists include collagen, thrombin and thromboxane 2. Thrombin is the most potent physiological activator of platelets. Weak agonists are ADP and epinephrine.

2. **A**

   The primary wave of aggregation in platelet aggregometry is caused by activation of the glycoprotein IIb/IIIa platelet membrane receptor. The secondary wave of aggregation is represented by platelet degranulation with recruitment of additional platelet aggregates.

3. **B**

   In response to the platelet agonists ADP and epinephrine, platelet aggregometry shows a biphasic pattern corresponding to primary and secondary waves of aggregation.

4. **E**

   Von Willebrand disease and Bernard-Soulier syndrome are similar in that only ristocetin induced aggregation will be affected. This is because ristocetin causes platelet agglutination through the VWF and gp1b-IX-V complex.

5. **B**

   Scott syndrome is a rare hemorrhagic bleeding disorder characterized by a defective scramblase mechanism that does not expose procoagulant phosphatidylserine to the outer surface of activated platelets. Consequently, coagulation factor complexes cannot assemble without binding to phosphatidylserine. There are no defects in platelet aggregation.

6. **C**

   Glanzmann thrombasthenia is a rare genetic disorder affecting the fibrinogen receptor α2β3. The defect can be quantitative or qualitative. Fibrinogen is required for normal platelet

   function, and without fibrinogen, platelets cannot aggregate. Therefore, in a platelet aggregation study, platelets would not aggregate to any of the agonists. Agglutination of platelets can, however, occur in response to ristocetin since fibrinogen is not required for the action of ristocetin.

7. **A**

   Striking abnormalities in the platelet aggregation study of answer A include the lack of the second wave of aggregation with ADP and decreased aggregation with epinephrine and collagen. This suggests deficiency of platelet granules or failure of granule release.

8. **C**

   Bernard-Soulier syndrome (BSS), also termed hemorrhagiparous thrombocytic dystrophy, is a hereditary bleeding disorder characterized by a deficiency or dysfunction of GP1b-V-IX. As a result, the only platelet agonist that would show a defect in aggregation would be ristocetin. Ristocetin causes agglutination through the VWF and GP1b-IX-V complex.

9. **C**

   The notable defects on platelet aggregation in a patient taking aspirin are absent aggregation with arachidonic acid, decreased aggregation with collagen and epinephrine and primary wave aggregation only with ADP.

10. **D**

    The k and α angle represent the rate of clot formation—the faster the rate of fibrin generation, the larger the angle. In hyperfibrinolysis, fibrinogen is broken down so k and α angle will decrease. The LY30 measures the decrease in pin amplitude oscillation 30 minutes after MA is reached and represents the rate of clot breakdown. Therefore, the LY30 would increase during hyperfibrinolysis.

The R parameter is the time from the start of the test to the time of initial fibrin formation. If there are clotting factor deficiencies, it would take longer to form the initial fibrin clot so R time would be prolonged.

The MA is the maximum amplitude of pin oscillation and measures the clot strength. The stronger the clot, the larger the MA. Platelets and fibrinogen are the major contributors to clot strength so thrombocytopenia would result in a decrease in MA.

11. A

The marked abnormality in this TEG is the low angle with normal R and MA. These findings are consistent with fibrinogen deficiency. Fibrinogen is required for platelet aggregation and for construction of the fibrin network. When fibrinogen is low, clot formation is slow, and this is reflected in the low angle and slightly prolonged K time.

12. C

The TEG is totally normal. Since coagulopathy is not present, this is most likely a surgical bleed.

13. A

Hyperfibrinolytic states occur when there is an increased activation of the fibrinolytic system, which results in or sustains bleeding. Primary fibrinolysis is characterized by excessive fibrinolytic activity that is not associated with thrombotic complications. This manifests on TEG as a reduction in the R-time, marked decrease in MA, CI <1.0 and a LY30 > 8%.

14. B

The euglobulin clot lysis time (ECLT) is an overall measure of fibrinolytic activity in plasma. To perform the test, venous blood is collected into chilled tubes containing trisodium citrate. After centrifuging, the plasma portion of the sample is collected and incubated with acetic acid. A precipitate forms, which is the euglobulin fraction containing, plasminogen, plasminogen activators and fibrinogen, while the supernatant is discarded. The euglobulin precipitate is redissolved in buffer and thrombin is added to form a clot. The time to clot lysis is variable from lab to lab, but for a reference range of 90–240 minutes, hyperfibrinolysis. occurs when the ECLT is less than 60 minutes and hypofibrinolysis occurs when the ECLT is > 240 minutes.

15. D

The urea clot lysis test is a qualitative Factor XIII screening assay that evaluates clot stability. A patient sample is mixed with either calcium or thrombin and the resulting clot is incubated in 5M urea (or 1% monochloracetic acid) for 24 hours. Only clots from Factor XIII-deficient individuals will dissolve.

16. B

In normal hemostasis, Factor XIII crosslinks antiplasmin to the fibrin strands, stabilizing the clot. However, if antiplasmin is deficient, the clot can be dissolved by plasmin, and a false positive result will occur.

If a Factor XIII deficient patient has been transfused plasma recently, this would result in a false negative in the clot lysis test since there will be some Factor XIII present in the transfused plasma.

Aminocaproic acid prevents fibrinolysis, which would again stabilize the clot.

The clot lysis test only detects the most severely affected Factor XIII-deficient homozygous patients with <2% Factor XIII activity.

17. B

The patient has an elevated PTT but normal PT. Further, the thrombin time was increased but reptilase time was normal. The blood sample used likely has heparin contamination, which would cause an elevation in the PTT but would have little effect on PT, if any. Heparin also increases thrombin time but has no effect on reptilase time.

18. C

The thrombin time measures the amount of time it takes for a plasma sample to clot after the addition of thrombin. Elevation of the thrombin time typically implies a quantitative or qualitative defect in fibrinogen. Reptilase time is a similar test except that thrombin is not used. Instead, reptilase, an enzyme derived from the snake Bothrops atrox, is used as a replacement for thrombin. Reptilase cleaves fibrinogen to release fibrinopeptide A only while thrombin releases both fibrinopeptides A and B. The thrombin time is influenced by heparin but reptilase time is not.

DIC would result in increases in both reptilase time and thrombin time.

19. A

A neonate may have elevated reptilase and thrombin times because neonatal fibrinogen differs from adult fibrinogen in its sialic acid content.

Warfarin would not affect TT or RT.

Direct thrombin inhibitors and heparin-like anticoagulants only increase TT.

20. A

Topical bovine thrombin is often contaminated with bovine Factor V. In this case, the patient developed an antibody to bovine Factor V, which cross-reacted with human Factor V. As Factor V decreased in the patient, PT and PTT increased along with bleeding. There have been many reports associated with factor inhibitor formation after the use of topical bovine thrombin.

21. D

The following tests are used to distinguish among the many types of Von Willebrand diseases based on quantitative versus qualitative measurements. Briefly, their function:

VWF:Ag (Von Willebrand Factor Antigen)–quantifies amount of VWF in plasma.

VWF:RCo (Von Willebrand Ristocetin Cofactor Activity)–the functional aspect of VWF is tested which measures the degree of platelet agglutination that occurs after the addition of ristocetin.

VWF:RCo/VWF:Ag ratio–if this value is > 0.6, most likely this will be type I VWD.

FVIII:C–functional FVIII coagulant assay

Multimers–the pattern of VWF multimers as viewed by electrophoresis

Ristocetin-induced platelet aggregation (RIPA)–measures the degree to which VWF binds to platelets with very low-dose ristocetin.

In type IIb VWD, there is a gain of function mutation wherein the GpIb binding region of VWF has enhanced binding for platelet receptor. Platelet binding to VWF can occur spontaneously in the circulation. Therefore, in type IIb VWD, there will be a unique finding in that RIPA will actually be increased. RIPA uses low concentrations of ristocetin that would not typically cause VWF binding and agglutination of platelet in normal persons.

In addition, both platelet and high molecular weight multimers will be cleared from the blood since the enhanced binding is selective for high molecular weight VWF multimers. As a result, HMW multimers will be decreased and thrombocytopenia will usually be seen in type IIb VWD.

22. A

Type IIa VWD is a qualitative defect characterized by defects of VWF that result in problems binding to platelet receptor GP1bα. In addition, high molecular weight (HMW) forms of VWF are either not formed or degraded prematurely in the plasma. Loss of HMW multimers with reduction (or normal) in RIPA differentiates type IIa from type IIb VWD. Type IIb VWD will have increased RIPA.

23. B

Type IIM VWD is a qualitative disorder similar to type IIb in that there is loss of function in VWF that is caused by mutations that disrupt VWF binding to platelets or subendothelium. However, it is differentiated from type IIb and type IIa by a normal multimeric distribution of VWF.

24. C

Type III VWD is a quantitative disorder resulting in virtually no circulating VWF. As a result, nothing will be seen in multimer electrophoresis; there will be no ristocetin-induced platelet aggregation, and VWF:Ag and VWF:RCo will be low to absent.

25. D

Type I VWD is a quantitative disorder resulting in mild to moderate reductions in VWF. As a result, the VWF:RCo and VWF:Ag would be decreased. Plasma levels of FVIII:C is reduced in proportion to VWF. Since VWF is functionally normal, the range of VWF multimers are also normal. The ratio of VWF:RCo;VWF:Ag is > 0.6.

26. A

The main laboratory abnormalities presenting in this bleeding patient with cancer is elevated D-dimer and FDP. In chronic DIC, there is persistent generation of thrombin from low-grade activation of coagulation factors. However, since there is only little ongoing consumption, often the platelets, PT, PTT and fibrinogen will be normal. Thrombin generation increases fibrin-degradation products (FDPs) through initiation of secondary fibrinolysis and generation of plasmin. To differentiate DIC from fibrinolysis, a more specific test like D-dimer is needed.

27. B

This patient has an isolated elevation in PTT along with spontaneous epistaxis. To determine whether the prolongation of PTT is due to factor deficiency or inhibitor, a PTT mixing study must be performed. In the PTT mixing study, patient plasma is mixed with normal plasma in a ratio of 1:1. If the mixture fails to correct, this is likely an inhibitor. However, if the PTT does correct, this is most likely a clotting factor deficiency.

28. D

Since the PTT corrected with the mixing study where a 1:1 ratio of patient plasma to normal plasma was used, this is a factor deficiency. All the other choices given would not have corrected.

29. C

This patient demonstrates easy and deep bruising with trauma. The platelet count and PT are normal, but PTT is elevated and corrects after 1:1 mixing study. This represents a factor deficiency. Hemophilia B is an X-linked recessive congenital deficiency of Factor IX.

30. B

Of these, aspirin use is the only one that would result in increased collagen-epinephrine closure time (CT) but normal collagen-ADP CT. The remaining choices would result in both increased collagen-EPI and collagen-ADP closure times.

31. A

Differentiating between these two entities is tricky because they have similar phenotypic parameters and clinical symptoms. Type 2B VWD has a defect in Von Willebrand factor, and pseudo platelet-type VWD has a defect in the platelet GP1b receptor. Both diseases lead to enhanced binding of platelets to VWF.

Ristocetin-induced agglutination of washed patient platelets mixed with normal plasma will show enhanced reactivity in platelet-type pseudo VWD but not in type 2B VWD.

32. D

The aPTT is performed by combining a surface activator (silica, kaolin, celite, ellagic acid, etc.), diluted phospholipid and calcium to citrated plasma. Then time to clot formation is measured. The PT is different in that it uses a combination of tissue factor, phospholipid and calcium.

33. C

Acute phase reactions that elevate Factor VIII levels can shorten the PTT. The remaining choices prolong the PTT.

34. A

The international normalized ratio (INR) is used to monitor warfarin therapy. The international sensitivity index (ISI) is given by the manufacturer to calculate the INR from the PT.

35. C

The activated clotting time is a point-of-care clotting test where whole blood is collected into a tube with a coagulation activator (kaolin, celite or glass particles) and magnetic stir bar. The time for clot formation is measured. It is used in situations where high-dose heparin therapy is needed like cardiopulmonary bypass. The aPTT becomes invalid in such cases.

36. B

The anti-Factor Xa assay is sometimes used to monitor low molecular weight heparin (LMWH) therapy since PTT cannot be used accurately.

37. D

The anti-Factor Xa assay is typically chromogenic but clotting-based assays are also available. In the chromogenic version, a standard curve is produced by combining known amounts of heparin to Factor Xa substrate with chromophore attached. The basic principle of the test is that Factor X cleaves the Factor Xa substrate, releasing chromophore and undergoing a color change that can be quantified. In a plasma sample with LMWH, antithrombin will promote Factor Xa inhibition and less Factor Xa will be available to cleave substrate. By comparing the results to the standard curve, the heparin concentration in the plasma can be calculated. Anti-Factor Xa assays are not affected by abnormal factor levels unlike the PTT. Ideally, they should be collected within 4 hours after administration of heparin.

The therapeutic range of unfractionated heparin for the treatment of DVT is 0.3–0.7 U/mL.

38. D.

A common screening assay for Factor V Leiden is the APC resistance assay. In this test, two aPTTs are run simultaneously–one with exogenous APC and one without APC. The ratio is simply the

APC-added aPTT divided by the APC-deficient aPTT. In a normal person, the addition of APC inactivates Factors Va and VIIIa, consequently prolonging the PTT. In contrast, a person with the Factor V Leiden mutation will not have as prolonged a clotting time. Thus, a normal patient will have a higher ratio compared to those with Factor V Leiden mutations.

39. A.

This patient does not have a Factor V Leiden mutation. Generally, APC resistance ratios > 2 are normal, between 1.5 and 2.0 are Factor V Leiden heterozygotes, and < 1.5 is typical of Factor V Leiden homozygotes. See answer 38 for how APC ratio is calculated.

40. C

The angle, MA and CI are all increased. The high angle represents rapid clot development, the high MA means strong clot development and the CI (Coagulation Index) is above 3. The CI is a mathematical formula determined by the manufacturer which is a combination of many values.

CI value > 3.0 suggests a hypercoagulable state whereas a CI < -3.0 suggests hypocoagulability.

41. C

Antithrombin normally inactivates Factor Xa and activated thrombin. In antithrombin deficiency, there is rapid thrombin generation, leading to faster overall clot development. The decrease in R with a CI > 3.0 represents an enzymatic hypercoagulability. Other diseases demonstrating enzymatic hypercoagulability include activated protein C resistance and a Factor V Leiden defect.

42. B

The serotonin release assay (SRA) represents the gold standard among all tests with a sensitivity and specificity reaching levels of 65% to > 90%.

43. D

Enzyme immunoassays for HIT typically have high negative predictive values (98–99%), but suffer from low positive predictive values because of detection of clinically insignificant anti-PF4-heparin antibodies. Heparin-treated patients who have anti-PF4-heparin antibodies rarely (2–15%) develop clinically evident HIT. Seroconversion after an initially negative test is almost always associated with clinically irrelevant antibodies.

44. C

Both factors in answers B and C increase the D-dimer level, accounting for its low specificity yet high sensitivity and negative predictive value for DVT exclusion.

The D-dimer is the degradation product of fibrin crosslinked by Factor XIII.

45. A

There are two classes of assays for detecting antiphospholipid antibodies: immunoassays and coagulation assays. The term "antiphospholipid antibodies" includes in its definition all of the antibodies detected by ELISA and lupus-anticoagulant assays.

The two immunoassays used for the detection of antiphospholipid antibodies are anti-β2-glycoprotein I and anticardiolipin IgG and IgM assays.

The dilute Russell viper venom test is a coagulation-based test to detect lupus anticoagulant.

46. D

The most sensitive test for the detection of antiphospholipid antibodies is the anticardiolipin IgG/IgM assay while lupus anticoagulant assays are the most specific but least sensitive.

47. B

There is already a strong clinical suspicion that this patient has antiphospholipid antibody syndrome based on recurrent spontaneous miscarriages and a prolonged PTT that fails to correct after a mixing study. Even though the screening test for (dRVVT) is negative, it is important to follow up with an immunoassay given the clinical suspicion of a thrombophilic disorder. Some patients do not test positive for lupus anticoagulant but have positive β2-GPI and/or anticardiolipin tests.

48. A

Platelets have alpha granules, delta (dense) granules, lysosomes and peroxisomes. Dense granules contain calcium, serotonin, adenine nucleotides (ATP, ADP), pyrophosphate and polyphosphate. Alpha granules are composed of many proteins including fibrinogen, fibronectin, VWF, P-selectin, osteonectin, VEGF, PDGF, TGF-β, thrombospondin, Factor V, multimerin, β-thromboglobulin, PF4, albumin, IgG, IgA and IgM, among others.

49. D

The gp IIb/IIIa complex (integrin α IIb β 3) is a major platelet membrane component whose activation initiates platelet aggregation and the formation of the primary platelet plug by binding to fibrinogen. The complex also binds to VWF, fibronectin and vitronectin.

Gp Ia/IIa and gp VI are collagen receptors.

The gpIb-IX-V binds to VWF.

50. B.

VWF can be found in Weibel-Palade bodies of endothelial cells, alpha granules of platelets, megakaryocytes and subendothelial connective tissue.

51. C

Endothelial cells play an important antithrombotic role by secreting prostaglandin I2 (prostacyclin) and NO. PI2 and NO both inhibit platelet aggregation. In addition, NO inhibits platelet adhesion to the vessel wall.

52. A

People with blood group O tend to have the lowest levels of VWF.

53. D

Wiskott-Aldrich syndrome is an X-linked disorder caused by mutations in the WAS gene. The defect may result in hemolytic anemia, immune thrombocytopenic purpura, neutropenia, arthritis and vasculitis of large and small vessels and damage to kidneys. Delta granules are always decreased, while the number of alpha granules varies.

Only alpha granules are reduced in Quebec syndrome and Gray Platelet syndrome.

Sebastian Anomaly is an autosomal dominant macrothrombocytopenia caused by mutations in the MYH9 gene.

Heparin-induced thrombocytopenia is caused by antibodies to the multimolecular complex of PF-4/heparin.

54. C

May-Hegglin anomaly, Epstein syndrome, Fechtner syndrome and Sebastian syndrome are autosomal dominant macrothrombocytopenias that are all part of a single disorder with a continuous clinical spectrum, ranging from sensorineural hearing loss, cataracts, nephritis and polymorphonuclear Dohle-like bodies. The common finding for all are mutations in the MYH9 gene encoding for the nonmuscle myosin heavy chain IIA (NMMHC-IIA).

Paris-Trousseau syndrome is caused by an 11q chromosome deletion resulting in congenital anomalies, a mild bleeding tendency, mental retardation, dysmegakaryopoiesis and platelet inclusion bodies.

55. C

Von Willebrand disease is the most common inherited bleeding disorder and has an estimated prevalence of 1% in the population.

56. D

All other types listed in this answer choice are inherited in an autosomal recessive fashion with the exception of type IIb VWD.

57. A

Type IIN VWD is characterized by a mutant form of VWF which has impaired binding to FVIII. Because of this defect, FVIII is markedly reduced in the circulation.

Answer (B) is a characteristic of type IIb VWD

Answer (C) is seen in type IIM VWD

Answer (D) is seen in type IIa VWD

58. B

Post-transfusion purpura is a rare cause of severe thrombocytopenia that typically occurs 5–12 days after transfusion. The mechanism of platelet destruction occurs through exposure and formation of antibodies to common platelet antigen, HPA-1a.

DIC is unlikely in this case since PT, PTT, fibrinogen and fibrin split products are normal. Hyperfibrinolysis is also unlikely since fibrinogen is normal

ITP is a diagnosis of exclusion, and thrombocytopenia often occurs after an infection.

59. A

Osler-Weber-Rendu syndrome, also known as hereditary hemorrhagic telangiectasia (HHT), is an autosomal dominant disorder with high penetrance. According to the Curacao criteria, an HHT diagnosis can be made if three out of four of the following criteria are met: epistaxis (spontaneous, recurrent), telangiectasias at multiple characteristic sites (lips, oral cavity, fingers, nose), visceral lesions (hepatic AVM, cerebral AVM, spinal AVM, pulmonary AVM, gastrointestinal telangiectasia), and a family history of a first-degree relative with HHT according to these criteria.

60. C

The lesion described in the vignette is a hemangioma. In infants, the combination of a vascular lesion, thrombocytopenia and coagulopathy is called Kasabach-Merrit syndrome (KMS). It is also known as hemangioma thrombocytopenia.

61. D

Childhood HUS is most commonly caused by *Escherichia coli* O157:H7, which produces Shiga toxins. It results in microangiopathic hemolytic anemia, thrombocytopenia and acute renal failure.

62. B

Although the classical pentad features of thrombotic thrombocytopenic purpura (TTP) include microangiopathic hemolytic anemia, thrombocytopenia, fever and neurological and renal abnormalities, this combination is not often seen in clinical practice. The cause of TTP is due to a deficiency of ADAMTS 13 protease (a disintegrin and metalloprotease with thrombospondin-1 like domains). Since ADAMTS 13 cleaves large Von Willebrand factor multimers, TTP results in abnormally large Von Willebrand factor multimers which strongly react with platelets and cause disseminated platelet thrombi.

63. D

Mutations in endoglin and ALK-1 are thought to be the major cause of Osler-Weber-Rendu syndrome, also known as HHT. The incidence has been reported as 1 in 5–8000. The earliest manifestations of the disease are nosebleeds, and adult HHT patient often exhibit an iron deficiency anemia.

64. C

Uremic platelet dysfunction is often falsely thought to be caused by increased uremia levels. However, there are multiple defects that contribute to uremic bleeding including intrinsic dysfunction of glycoprotein IIb/IIIa, decreased prostaglandin metabolism, decreased platelet thromboxane A2 generation, abnormal platelet-vessel wall interactions and reduction in intracellular ADP and serotonin. Uremic toxins such as guanidinosuccinic acid and methylguanidine are potential contributors to platelet dysfunction, likely through stimulation of NO production.

Elevations in blood urea nitrogen (BUN) and serum creatinine have no correlation with bleeding risk.

Patients with familial azotemia, an autosomal dominant disorder resulting in high plasma urea levels, have normal in vitro platelet function.

65. A

The platelet "function defect" associated with cardiopulmonary bypass is not an intrinsic defect. It occurs because the heparin used during bypass results in inhibition of endogenous thrombin. Without thrombin, platelets are not activatable.

66. C

The acronym CATCH-22 makes it simple to remember DiGeorge and velocardiofacial syndromes with *c*ardiac *a*bnormalities, *T*-cell deficit, *c*left palate and *h*ypocalcemia due to a chromosome 22 deletion. Aside from the congenital abnormalities, these syndromes are known to cause a mild macrothromboctyopenia.

67. A

Platelet-type disorders will generally manifest as mucosal bleeding (petechiae, purpura), moderate bleeding from small wounds and heavy menses. The remaining answer choices represent physical findings caused by coagulation disorders.

68. D

The two drugs that block the ADP receptor on platelets are ticlopidine and clopidogrel.

Answer choices A and B are GPIIb/IIIa receptor antagonists.

Dipyridamole inhibits phosphodiesterase, increasing the levels of cAMP and cGMP and reversibly inhibits platelet aggregation.

69. A

Vitamin K-dependent factors in the clotting system include Factors II, VII, IX and X, and proteins C and S. Vitamin K is needed for a gamma-carboxylation reaction that occurs on each of these proteins' glutamic acid residues, which allows these proteins to bind to phospholipid and cell membranes.

70. D

The factors that make up the intrinsic pathway are Factors VIII, IX, XI and XII. Answer choice (A) is the vitamin K-dependent clotting factors. The extrinsic coagulation system consists of Factor VII and tissue factor (Answer B). Answer (C) is the common factor pathway.

71. B

Acquired Factor X deficiency classically occurs in amyloidosis and is thought to occur from adsorption of Factor X to amyloid fibrils.

71. C

Factor VII has the shortest in vivo plasma half-life at around 5 hours.

73. B

Factor XIII has the longest in vivo plasma half-life at around 200 hours.

74. D

Protein S decreases during a thrombotic event. That is why it is important to perform testing for protein S at least 10 days after the event.

Protein S is lower in women than in men.

Protein S is low at birth but increases to normal range by 6 months of age.

Oral contraceptives, estrogen use, warfarin and vitamin K all decrease the level of protein S.

75. C

Protein S exists in the body in two forms: free and bound. Normally, 40% is found free in plasma and the remaining 60% is complexed to C4bBP. In acute phase reactions, C4bBP becomes elevated and binds to and reduces circulating protein S. This makes it appear that there is a protein S deficiency.

76. A

In familial C4bBP deficiency, free protein S is increased because there is no C4bBP to bind to. This increase in free protein S, however, does not have an increased predilection for bleeding.

Pregnancy, DIC, liver failure and nephrotic syndrome are all causes of decreased protein S levels.

77. C.

Severe prekallikrein deficiency is a rare autosomal trait disorder which often presents as an incidental prolongation of the PTT in a person without a history of excessive bleeding. The PTT may be shortened by longer incubation time with the contact reagent as this gives enough time for Factor XII to activate through prekallikrein-independent mechanisms. None of the remaining choices will correct with prolonged incubation times.

78. A.

An incidentally prolonged PTT without history of bleeding can be seen in high molecular weight kininogen (HMWK) deficiency, prekallikrein deficiency and Factor XII deficiency. If the patient had reported a history of excessive bleeding, then one would consider deficiencies in Factors VIII, IX or XI since these would cause abnormal hemostasis. Low molecular weight kininogen does not play a role in coagulation in vitro. HMWK deficiency (also known as Fitzgerald trait, Williams trait and Flaujeac trait) is inherited in an autosomal recessive fashion. A definitive diagnosis is established by using high molecular weight kininogen deficient plasma.

79. B

Factor VII deficiency is a rare autosomal recessive disorder that typically results in a bleeding diathesis. However, it may also be associated with thrombosis. Only the PT is prolonged in Factor VII deficiency. The treatment of choice for bleeding in a Factor VII-deficient patient is recombinant human-activated Factor VIIa.

80. D

The incidence of DIC in severe infection and sepsis has been reported at 58–83%. Another disease with a high incidence of DIC is acute promyelocytic leukemia.

81. B

DIC is characterized by the systemic activation of coagulation resulting in consumption of all coagulation proteins (antithrombin included) and platelets. Bacterial infection induces coagulation directly via induction of tissue factor on endothelial cells and mononuclear cells. Fibrin-degradation products would be increased in DIC.

Factor VIIa is thought to be the central mediator of DIC in sepsis.

82. A

Congenital dysfibrinogenemia is an autosomal dominant trait usually caused by a missense mutation in any of the three fibrinogen genes, α (FGA), β(FGB) or γ (FGG). Laboratory abnormalities will result in increased PT, PTT and thrombin times due to disruption in the common pathway. There can be either bleeding or thrombosis but this is not common as nearly 55% have no symptoms.

83. D

Both Hemophilia A and B are X-linked recessive disorders. Hemophilia B results in deficiency of coagulation Factor IX.

84. B

Heparin inhibits thrombin and Factor Xa indirectly by binding to and enhancing the activity of antithrombin.

85. A

Apixaban and rivaroxaban are direct Xa inhibitors. Bivalirudin and dabigatran are direct thrombin inhibitor.

LMWH interact with antithrombin to inactivate XA and thrombin

86. B

Heparin-induced thrombocytopenia (HIT) is a challenging clinical and laboratory diagnosis. The typical course in heparin naïve patients is a platelet count drop of >50% or <150 × 10^9/L beginning 5–14 days after heparin exposure. Thrombocytopenia may be isolated or in conjunction with arterial and/or venous thrombosis. HIT is caused by antibodies to a multimolecular complex of heparin (H) and platelet Factor 4 (PF4). The apparent paradox of thrombocytopenia with thrombosis is thought to be caused by thrombin generation and procoagulant microparticle release when the PF4/H complex binds to platelet and monocyte Fc receptors.

In this patient, physical examination did not exhibit splenomegaly so (A) is incorrect.

Antibodies to HPA-1a occur in post-transfusion purpura to multiparous women or those with previous transfusions. However, the platelet count

typically drops to less than 10 ×10^9/L and bleeding often occurs. Thus (C) is incorrect.

The coagulation profile is relatively normal in this patient with the exception of D-dimer, and no schistocytes were present on the peripheral blood smear, thus ruling out DIC (answer D).

Mechanical destruction of platelets from the cardiopulmonary bypass circuit typically occurs intraoperatively and reaches the platelet nadir by the second or third day after surgery (answer E)

87. A, C, E

The incidence of PF4-heparin antibodies in patients undergoing orthopedic surgery is 14%, but the actual incidence of HIT in this patient population is 3–5%. Low molecular weight heparin (LMWH) has been reported to have a 5–10-fold lower risk of HIT than unfractionated heparin (UFH).

Female gender has been associated with an odds ratio of 2.37 of developing HIT. The incidence of HIT is quite low – less than 1% in those undergoing chronic hemodialysis

88. A

PF4 is a cationic, 7.8 kDa protein that is released from the alpha granules of activated platelets as a complex with a chondroitin sulfate proteoglycan carrier.

89. D

Warfarin and phenprocoumon are vitamin K antagonists that should not be given in patients with acute HIT because they decrease the level of proteins C and S, which can increase the risk of venous limb gangrene. Abciximab is a glycoprotein IIb/IIIa inhibitor, and has no role in anticoagulation in a patient with HIT. Suitable alternatives include direct thrombin inhibitors, danaproid (an antithrombin-dependent Factor Xa inhibitor) and fondaparinux (a low molecular weight heparin).

90. C

This vignette depicts the classical findings of Trousseau's syndrome–recurrent, migratory venous thromboses preventable by anticoagulation therapy with heparin but not with warfarin. Thrombotic events typically appear before a tumor would otherwise be detected, therefore, the clinician should focus on investigating an occult malignancy. Although the mechanism is not fully understood, it is thought that tumor cells secrete cell-derived tissue factor.

91. A

Normally, activated protein C degrades Factors Va and VIIIa at specific arginine residues; however, in activated protein C resistance, Factor V contains a point mutation which renders it resistant to degradation by activated protein C. This defect is known as Factor V Leiden, which occurs in more than 95% of cases and is caused by a point mutation at one of the three arginine cleavage sites in the Factor V gene.

92. D

Factor V Leiden is the most common genetic cause of venous thromboembolism.

93. E

Homocysteinemia is the only one of the listed disorders that is inherited in an autosomal recessive fashion. The remainder of the disorders are autosomal dominant.

94. B

The Prothrombin Gene G20210A mutation occurs rarely in nonwhite populations and the highest prevalence is seen in Southern European populations. The occurrence of double heterozygosity of the prothrombin mutation and Factor V Leiden increases the thrombotic risk 3–5-fold above the risk of a single defect.

Although close to 87% of patients with the prothrombin mutation have high plasma prothrombin values, plasma prothrombin concentrations cannot be used to screen for the prothrombin gene mutation since there is significant overlap.

95. C

APS is a prothrombotic disorder that affects both venous and arterial systems. The most common site for venous thrombosis is in the deep veins of the lower limbs, while the most common site for arterial thrombosis is the cerebral arterial circulation. Only a small subgroup of patients develop catastrophic antiphospholipid syndrome where clots in multiple vascular beds leads to multi-organ failure and death. The diagnosis of APS requires at least one clinical and one laboratory criterion each.

96. A

Elevated levels of homocysteine may be acquired or hereditary. The hereditary causes include mutations in either cystathionine-β-synthase (CBS) or MTHFR. Mutations in MTHFR can lead to increased homocysteine levels but rarely result in homocysteine levels that overflow into the urine (homocystinuria). On the basis of retrospective control studies, there is an association with increased risk of arterial and venous thrombosis and elevations in homocysteine. Homozygosity for C677T mutations in the MTHFR gene is not an independent risk factor for arterial or venous thrombosis.

97. C

Plasminogen activator inhibitor-1 (PAI-1) is a serine protease inhibitor which blocks the activity of t-PA and u-PA to convert plasminogen to plasmin, thereby inhibiting fibrinolysis.

α2-antiplasmin is responsible for inactivating plasmin.

Thrombin-activatable fibrinolysis inhibitor (TAFI) suppresses fibrinolysis by the removal of lysine residues from the fibrin clot, which prevents binding of plasminogen and t-PA to the fibrin clot.

Tissue Factor Pathway Inhibitor (TFPI) is an anticoagulation protein which binds to TF/FVIIa complex and by directly inhibiting FXa as well.

98. D

Antifibrinolytics such as aminocaproic acid and tranexamic acid are the best treatment choices during primary hyperfibrinolysis. They inhibit fibrinolysis by inhibiting the conversion of plasminogen to the fibrinolytic enzyme plasmin. It is very important to distinguish primary fibrinolysis from disseminated vascular coagulation (DIC) since antifibrinolytics are dangerous to use in DIC and could cause disseminated thrombosis.

99. A

There is increased fibrinolytic activity in the endometrium of women with an IUD associated with menorrhagia, which can be treated with antifibrinolytic agents.

In severe trauma patients, a greater degree of hyperfibrinolysis confers a greater risk of death.

The fibrinolysis that may occur during OLT results in increased plasma t-PA, decreased fibrinogen and α2-antiplasmin, and elevated degradation products.

Patients with amyloidosis and hyperfibrinolysis usually respond well to antifibrinolytic therapy.

100. A

Type 1 plasminogen deficiency is a quantitative disorder while type 2 plasminogen deficiency is a qualitative disorder. Ligneous conjunctivitis is a common manifestation of type 1 plasminogen deficiency. Pseudomembranes tend to form on the upper eyelid because there is a low level of plasminogen that is incapable of breaking down the accumulation of fibrin-rich tissue. Despite having decreased plasminogen, there is no increased risk of thrombosis. Therefore, the 2001 CAP Consensus Conference recommended excluding plasminogen activity or antigen measurements in thrombophilia workups.

Index

Printed in the United States
By Bookmasters